SUPERNATURAL HEALING,
SUPER PRACTICAL HEALTH,

OILS

OF THE

BIBLE

AND YOU!

ANDREW EDWIN JENKINS

WORKSHOP
EDITION!

Supernatural Healing, Super Practical Health, Oils of the Bible, and You! Copyright 2018, Overflow, LLC.

Adapted from *The Field Guide to Healing*- Copyright 2016, Overflow, LLC. All right reserved. No part of this book may be reproduced in any form or by any means without permission in writing by the publisher.

For more information about future events go to www.WeOverflow.com/Healing.

For more information about content in the book, go to www.OverflowFaith.com

ISBN 13: 978-1985144262

ISBN 10: 1985144263

Connect online!

Podcast-
Jenkins.tv

Social-
www.Facebook.com/AndrewEJenkins
www.Facebook.com/WeOverflow
www.Instagram.com/AndrewEJenkins
www.Twitter.com/AndrewEJenkins

YouTube-
www.YouTube.com/Overflow

Website-
www.OverflowFaith.com
www.Overflow.org

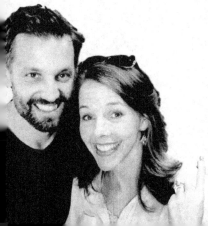

#OVER*flow*

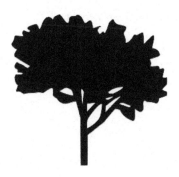

Contents

AN OVERVIEW OF WHERE WE'RE HEADED!

Intro: The Big Idea

WHERE ELSE WOULD YOU GO FOR LIFE?

Just a few years ago I was stressed out, overweight, pulling 80-hour work weeks, and aging way too fast. The constant stress of leading a church, a nonprofit, and being a husband and father kept me moving fast. The days seemed long, yet the weeks seemed short. Incredibly short.

I remember looking across the bed more than once and asking Cristy, as I fell asleep for the night, "Is it really *already* Thursday? Another week almost gone... *really*?"

Most of those conversations were smattered with questions about finances. We were living paycheck to paycheck. Barely. Most weeks consisted of transferring money right back out of savings that we'd just put in. Even at that, we were deciding if it was more important to pay the power bill or put

I WASN'T REALLY EXPERIENCING ANY OF THE THREE THINGS JOHN PRAYED ABOUT!

gas in the car this week. Don't get me wrong: everything was always paid. But it didn't seem like we were living the abundant life. I was tired, I was unhealthy, and we were just scraping by.

During this season, I remembered the words the Apostle John prayed for the church when he was older. He blessed the church, saying, "I pray that you may prosper in all things and be in health, just as your soul prospers" (3 John 2 NKJV).

Right there, he assumed Jesus' followers were...

- Prospering in "all things" (maybe the topic of another book, OK?)

- Experiencing physical health

- Enjoying vitality of the soul

I wasn't really experiencing *any* of the three things John prayed about!

Just how bad it was...

A few years ago Cristy began building a business in the health and wellness industry, working from home.[1] I didn't pay much attention to what she was doing until she won an all-expenses paid trip for two to Hawaii. Then, she had my attention!

We stayed in a great hotel while on the trip- five stars! And, we had a full length mirror in the bathroom- something we don't have at home. Its reflection gave me the first full length glimpse of myself I'd seen in over a decade. As I looked at my reflection, I noticed that I didn't quite look the same as I used to...

I asked my wife about it- in the form of a statement. "I've gained a little weight, haven't I?"

She *sweetly* told me I "could stand" to lose a little bit of weight. I could tell she didn't really want to be direct about it, because she didn't want to crush my pride. So, that's how she phrased it: *I could stand to...*

---

[1] Go to www.HowWeDoIt.info for more info on her business.

"Like how much?" I asked. Then, I tried to quantify it before she could answer: "Maybe 10 pounds or so?"

She gave me a polite, sing-song "Hmmm" and suggested I move my number higher.

"20 pounds?" I replied.

She looked at me and smiled. She motioned that I should go to *another* higher number.

"*25?*" I asked, slightly elevating the pitch of my voice, to accentuate the five and the finality of the number. I knew I had *some* to lose, but her number was a bit higher than I actually thought...

She motioned a bit higher...

"30?"

"Yeah, probably so," she told me. "You could do at least twenty five..." (At least? I thought.) "...but probably closer to 30 would do it."

> THROUGHOUT SCRIPTURE, PHYSICAL HEALTH ISN'T SEPARATED FROM SPIRITUAL VITALITY.

I started running the numbers in my head, thinking how impossible it would be to get to where I needed to be. How long it would take...

In the end, I lost 50 pounds. And as I did, everything began to change...

Big changes

As we walked along the beach in Hawaii on that trip, I told Cristy I would help her with her business when we got back home. And I did.

I jumped into two things immediately. First, I began losing the weight and getting healthy. Right now, I'm in better shape than I've ever been in my life. And, I'm happy to say that I became the family guinea pig / crash test dummy for a lot of the amazing products she has in her wellness business.

Second, I began helping her teach. Sometimes that took the form of writing books and training manuals and blog posts; other times it took the form of shooting videos; many times it took the form of taking the stage and talking to others live. However, the common thread with all of it was business. In a real way, I took the gifts I'd been given (teaching, communicating) and simply used them within the existing business model. And I simply taught others about *business* when I did.

Somehow, I never connected the dots that perhaps I should teach about the healing journey I was on. Or the things about Divine healing I already knew from my days working in a church, in a nonprofit, and teaching the Bible in various venues. It never dawned on me that others might actually desire to take a similar journey themselves. Or that they may feel a hunger to lead others down that same path.

It's really somewhat odd that I missed it. Again, I've taught *healing* before. I've prayed for others to be healed- and they were. I taught my former staff and interns to pray for healing. In fact, we've taught our kids how to pray for others in this way- and seen results.

> IT NEVER DAWNED ON ME THAT OTHERS MIGHT WANT TO TAKE A SIMILAR JOURNEY THEMSELVES.

Remind me to tell you about the time that Ivey (then 7) prayed for someone to be healed of cancer- and they were! Then, when we were telling the story to a kind woman, she asked us to pray for her because she had the same cancer, so Ivey did and saw that woman healed as well!

You're still the same person

As I made these changes, I began looking through the Bible- even though I wasn't yet teaching it to a wider audience. I found that throughout Scripture, *physical health isn't separated from spiritual vitality*. They're inextricably linked together. This means if you're excelling in one and floundering in the other, you could probably excel even *more* in the one!

Anyway, when people had an ailment in the Old Testament, they were instructed to go to the priests. One pastor writes, "If someone had leprosy and later said they were clean, to whom were they sent to determine if they were healed? The priest!"

When Jesus healed lepers... even He sent the healed person to the priest (Matthew 8:4, Luke 17:14).

In the New Testament, the concept is the same: "The New Testament says, if there be any sick among you, call who? The elders of the church" (see James 5:14).[2] And it's not because they didn't have doctors. In fact, a well-known physician named Luke wrote *more* of the New Testament than anyone else- including Paul. Yes, Paul wrote more books, but Luke's self-titled Gospel and his Book of Acts boast more words and pages than all of Paul's letters combined!

Whereas we compartmentalize our lives- and think *this* is spiritual, *that* is physical, *this* is sacred, *that* is secular- we're always the same person. And our bodies *and* our spirits *and* our souls are all part of who we are.

> "NOT EVEN A FRACTION OF A PERCENTAGE INCLUDED A PASTOR, CHURCH, BIBLE, OR GOD..."

Think about it this way: a *USA Today* article asked people plainly in a poll: "Where do you go when you're sick?"

The results were what you might expect to see:

- 50% call their primary care physician

- 31% rely on what they see in the media

- 5% talk to a relative or friend

- 5% consult self-help books

- 4% learn in school courses

- 2% talk to their pharmacist

---

[2] Henry Wright, *A More Excellent Way*, p7.

I know... that doesn't add up to 100%. None of the remaining responses didn't amount to a full percentage point. This means that "not even a fraction of a percentage included a pastor, church, Bible, or God..."[3]

Is that odd to you that no one sought the true source of all healing?

Now, I'm *pro*-doctors. We've birthed several of our kids at the hospital (and a few at home!). We've put two kids in casts in the past twelve months (a gymnastic accident and a playground mishap resulted in two broken arms!). Just last week we ran to the ER for an X-ray after a zip-line accident in the backyard. We've also sought the help of other professionals to help with some of the issues we've had with adopted sons.

At the same time, I don't think everything for which people in our culture seek medical attention is necessarily a medical issue. And, even when it is, it's often for something that could be- *dare I say it?*- cured in a more natural way.

Where I am today

Let me disclose two of my presuppositions. I believe that, first of all, we can experience God's supernatural power *now*. The same power that raised Jesus from the dead now resides in you and gives life to your body (Romans 8:11). Maybe we should tap into that.

Second, my experience suggests that many of the issues we deal with have spiritual and emotional roots. I'm not saying that if you sin God will curse you with sickness- *not at all!* In fact, we'll deal with that misnomer early in this book. However, if the deepest

> "I WILL SEEK WHAT WAS LOST AND BRING BACK WHAT WAS DRIVEN AWAY, BIND UP THE BROKEN AND STRENGTHEN WHAT WAS SICK."

and richest part of us is the spirit inside, doesn't it make sense that the condition of our soul might effect our entire being? Remember what John wrote- he prayed people would prosper in "all things" and in "health" to the degree their souls were vibrant and alive (3 John 2)?

---

[3] *A More Excellent Way*, p69.

If this the case, if even *some* of the issues we face our spiritual in nature, then "we have asked the medical community to do something they are not qualified to do- to pastor us and deal with spiritual issues."[4] Incidentally, it's probably not just "some" of our issues that are related to the care of our souls- it's probably *many*.

I saw this in my past career, helping drug addicts. Most of the *physical* issues they wrestled with were related to a lack of identity, feelings of unforgiveness, and wounds and lies they were believing. Get that: spiritual and emotional issues had become physical.[5]

Throughout my experience in "church world" things were no different. Many times- *not always, but often-* there were underlying issues that were simply surfacing as physical problems. The bad news is that this is hard to hear when someone is suggesting that this might be *your* problem; the good news is that its extremely easy to deal with once you do hear it!

Where are those skilled to heal?

The prophet Ezekiel rebuked the spiritual leaders of his day: "The weak you have not strengthened, nor have you healed those who were sick, nor bound up the broken..." (34:4). The spiritual leaders weren't supposed to just teach people information about God; they were supposed to help people encounter Him and experience the riches of His Kingdom- *including health*. When they didn't do this, God Himself promised, "I will seek what was lost and bring back what was driven away, bind up the broken and strengthen what was sick" (34:16).

Of course, Jeremiah explained *how* God planned to do this: "I will give you shepherds according to My heart" (3:15). That is, His plan to heal His people was not a world-class HMO or better health insurance for everyone; His plan was- *and remains-* to send shepherds to His people who will express His heart to them in such a way that they are healed.

---

[4] *A More Excellent Way*, p69.

[5] You'll understand why, once you see how the limbic system works.

Paul prayed that "the God of peace Himself sanctify you completely; and may your whole spirit, soul, and body be preserved blameless..." (1 Thessalonians 5:23 NKJV). In other words, the same God who revives your spirit also brings total healing to your mind, emotions, and body. And, when He does His work He most often does it through people. He literally uses His people to express and demonstrate His power!

Isaiah wrote of days that were coming when people who died at 100 years old would be considered "accursed" for dying young (see Isaiah 65:20). It all makes me wonder if maybe we've missed something... if maybe we need to find those who are skilled to heal today.

What if...?

I was running early one morning while it was still dark- and praying. At the same time. That's kinda what you do when you have 9 kids in the house.

"Call Pastor Rick," the Lord told me. I didn't make any logical sense that I would call him- I had no "transactional" reason to do so, even though I've always felt a spiritual connection to him.

I called him later that same day. Turns out, he'd just used some material I'd written about prayer at a conference a few weeks prior. He meant to give me a call, too, but hadn't gotten around to it...

We met for lunch a few days later and I told him I was looking to teach about healing again- but to do so in a more comprehensive way. To do it in a way that you'll find in this book. A way that invites- and expects- the miraculous to happen. A way that also realizes that we're created to "choose life" and walk in health and wellness as a lifestyle. A way that looks at what the authors of the Bible assumed we might understand and unpacks it...

"When do you want to teach it at my church?" he asked. It was almost like he was ready before I was. So, I began writing and we began scheduling...

Then a few weeks later I reconnected with a friend of mine, Mayer, via Facebook. He leads the small groups and discipleship ministry at Word Alive- the church where my friend Kent Mattox pastors. Kent and Mayer had asked each other about me a few days before we connected. Turns out, Kent's Twitter account was "malfunctioning." Every time someone retweeted Kent, my name popped up on his phone. You'll read a little about Kent later in the book.[6]

We hadn't seen each other in a few years, so Mayer, Kent, and I decided to grab lunch. "How long would it take you to be ready to teach this?" Kent asked. Then- "And how many weeks do you need?" He asked if I was available to come to their studio and shoot a few shows.

Time to surf

I knew the Lord had sent a huge wave and it was time to surf. That was a message the Lord sent to me during the middle of all of this...

The previous Fall, I'd gone surfing with my friend Scott while leading a men's weekend event in San Diego.[7] A professional, he took me to the beach where we stood on the sand and watched the waves for a few minutes. While ashore, he taught me how to surf by showing me how to position myself on the board and then jump to my feet once the wave began propelling me. Next, we paddled out, side-by-side. As the first wave approached- one I would never have taken- Scott spun my board around, pushed it gently with the wave, and sent me on my way. I surfed the first time I ever tried. I didn't create the wave. I didn't rush to catch it. I didn't even have a board. I was simply nudged into what was already happening.

I don't know about you, but I've tried to create waves before. I've tried to "figure things out" (who can logically figure out a wave?), I've tried to create momentum (really- create a wave?), and I've worked really hard (but you don't work hard to ride a wave- you just hop on it and allow it to do the work *for* you, don't you?!). (By the way, during that unhealthy, overworked season, *I was really trying...* on all fronts!)

---

[6] You'll meet Kent later in the book. The question I asked- and the answer he gave- will astound you!

[7] Go to www.EatSleepAdvance.com for more info on that event and future events.

Where are you?

Maybe you're where I was just a few years ago. Maybe you need a miracle, maybe you don't. I didn't realize how drained and tired I was… until I was actually healthy and well.

What if you just feel stuck? What if you find yourself tolerating physical nuisances which you know aren't part of the abundant life- things like restless sleep, etc., etc., blah, blah, blah? Do you just "throw in the towel" because the miracle is out of reach? Or is there another way, a way that Jesus taught all along…?

If you're tired and weary, this book is for you. Or if you know people who are tired and weary, and you feel called to love them- or lead them- then welcome. Maybe this is your wave, too.

What you'll find

In the next chapter I'll introduce you to the 3 habits: *think*, *touch*, and *tell*. I'll explain them, briefly, before we work through each one in detail over the course of the book. If you can remember those three words, you can- *I guaranteed you*- bless anyone with the concepts I'll teach you.

First, work your way through each chapter in order. You'll learn about *think* in chapter 2, *touch* in chapters 3 & 4, and *tell* in chapter 5. We'll review them together in chapter 6, then I'll give you a step-by-step ministry model in chapter 7.

Second, take time to answer the questions which follow each chapter. They will help you refine what you learned in the previous chapter.

Third, look to the online resources for more help. You'll find hours of video teaching, graphics you can use for quick reference, and other bonus materials at OverflowFaith.com.

As always, thank you for joining me on this journey.

THE BIG IDEA

#Overflow,

[signature: Andrew]

Andrew Edwin Jenkins

AJ@overflow.org

Revised February 2018

PS- Let me clarify how I use the terms *healing* and *health* throughout this book...

When I refer to *healing*, I'm denoting something that God does. When I refer to *health*, I'm referencing something we do- choices we make. I know, there's not really a "cut and dry" line between the two. In fact, as you read on you'll see that these two actually work together, enhancing each other.

Oh... the term *healing*... you'll learn that this one is often referred to in the Bible as *iaomai*. And the word *health*... *therapeuo*. More on that in a few pages.

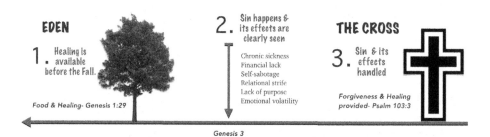

Notice that healing is present in the very beginning- before sin happens (1).

When sin occurs, we see the fruit of it- sickness, lack, strife, lack of purpose, emotional volatility (2) (These are the fruits of bad roots you will see later in the book). We see this bad fruit beginning in Genesis 3 and weaving its way throughout the Bible.

Jesus deals with sin on the Cross (3). He restores relational intimacy and physical health (3).

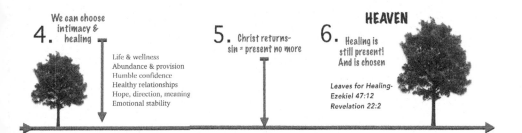

4. We can choose intimacy & healing

Life & wellness
Abundance & provision
Humble confidence
Healthy relationships
Hope, direction, meaning
Emotional stability

5. Christ returns- sin = present no more

6. HEAVEN
Healing is still present! And is chosen

Leaves for Healing-
Ezekiel 47:12
Revelation 22:2

We can now choose to walk in both intimacy & health (4). Good fruits can emerge.

Jesus will return at some point in the future (5), and sin will no longer exist (nothing impure is in Heaven- Revelation 21:27; all things are new- Revelation 21:5; people insistent to sin are not there- Revelation 21:8).

Notice, though, the opportunity to choose healing will (6).

This leads me to believe that we were created to choose wellness AND intimacy. Both were our origin in Eden; both are our destiny in Heaven. The presence of the Kingdom in the New Testament always includes both.

THE BIG IDEA

1. The 3 Habits

INTRODUCING THE HABITS TO WALK IN WHOLENESS & HEALING

"...On either side of the river was the tree of life, bearing twelve kinds of fruit, yielding its fruit every month; and the leaves of the tree were for the healing of the nations" (Revelation 22:2 NIV).

A. Healing happens in ___Heaven___. When healing occurs we witness the presence of the future.

- Physical healing- and physical health- demonstrates the presence of the Kingdom.[8]

- This healing existed before sin- and continues eternally.

---

[8] Catch this- even health demonstrates the presence of the Kingdom. This is a major point you'll see throughout this book.

1. When we see healing manifest on earth, we're actually seeing __**Heaven** **coming** **down**__, breaking into the world in which we live.

- **Jesus told the disciples to tell people the Kingdom of God had come near when they healed them** (Matthew 10:7, Luke 10:9).

- He Himself said that when He drove out demons, **it was a sign that the Kingdom was present** (Matthew 12:28, Luke 11:20).

2. The prophet Ezekiel & the apostle John learned something interesting when they saw the __**tree** **of** **life**__ in Heaven.

- "On each side of the river stood the tree of life... **And the leaves of the tree are for the healing of the nations**" (Revelation 22:2 NIV).[9]

- "Fruit trees of all kinds will grow on both banks of the river. Their leaves will not wither, nor will their fruit fail. Every month they will bear fruit, because the water from the sanctuary flows to them. **Their fruit will serve for food and their leaves for healing**" (Ezekiel 47:12 NIV).

- Whereas most people think about the tree of life- and its presence in Heaven- in *symbolic* terms, simply *spiritualizing* it, we need to remember that **the first time we see the tree in Genesis it is an actual tree in the *physical* world.** Adam and Eve could have eaten its fruit. They could have climbed this tree or sat in its shade. It wasn't symbolic; it was *real*.

---

[9] The word for "healing" here is *therapeuo*. We'll learn more about the word later. For now, think about this: *Why is there healing in Heaven?*

3. Jesus always asked people if they wanted to experience the presence of the __Kingdom__ - the implication might be that some people __don't__, that they prefer their __old identity__.

- He asked the blind man, **"What do you want me to do for you?"** (see Mark 10:51). The answer might *seem* obvious; but Jesus asked for certainty.

- He asked the invalid at the Pool of Bethesda, **"Do you want to be made well...?"** (John 5:6). The implication is that some people don't want to be.

- **We must be willing to receive the identify of Heaven, as sons and daughters.** As odd as it sounds, sometimes it's difficult to let go of the old identity.

B. __Healing__ & __wholeness__ were present in the beginning, before sin. __Health__ & __wellness__ were not results of the chaos created by the fall. __Healing__ & __wholeness__ already existed.

- **A moment ago I suggested healing shows us the presence of the future.**

- **Healing also shows us the reality of our past.**

1. In Eden, God gave every plant for food- and __more__!

- Genesis 1:29-30 reads, "Then God said, 'I give you every seed-bearing plant on the face of the whole earth and every tree that has fruit with seed in it. **They will be yours for food.** And to all the beasts of the earth and all the birds in the sky and all the creatures that move along the ground—everything that has the breath of life in it—I give every green plant for food.' And it was so" (NIV).

- **The Hebrew word used here, which we translate as "food," is *oklah*.**[10]

> OKLAH INCLUDES THE THINGS YOU EAT, BUT IT IS MORE. OKLAH INCLUDES MEDICINES.

  - *Oklah* includes the things you eat, but it is more. *Oklah* includes medicines. Notice, these were here in the beginning.

  - We see the same word used in Ezekiel 47:12 (see the previous page). The word *oklah*, in both instances, would include herbs, teas, and other plant-based products.

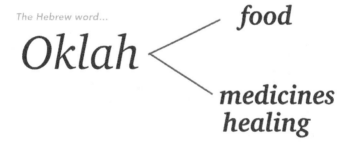

  - **"...the plant kingdom offers countless varieties of medicines created by God- sufficient to address every ailment known to humankind.** Instead of spending billions on secular profit-motivated research to create new synthetic

---

[10] The Old Testament was originally penned in Hebrew.

drugs, antibiotics, vaccines, and surgical procedures, our research should be towards discovering, studying, and applying the vast array of medicines that God has already perfected in forms already available to us."[11]

- **"Let your food be your medicine and your medicine be your food"** (Hippocrates).

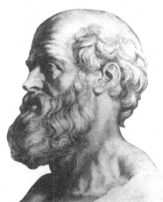

66

LET YOUR FOOD BE YOUR MEDICINE AND YOUR MEDICINE BE YOUR FOOD...

— Hippocrates

99

2. Why was __*healing*__ and __*wholeness*__ available in the Garden before sin (especially if sickness is a result of the Fall)? And why is it present in Heaven?

- **We were created to *choose* wellness, just like we were created to *choose* intimacy.** In fact, I believe we will want to choose wellness when we walk fully in who we were designed by God to be.

---

[11] David Stewart, *Healing Oils of the Bible*, p165. We will discuss pharmaceuticals in more detail, when we talk about Habit 2: Touch.

- "God's perfect will is not to heal you; His perfect will is that you don't get sick."[12]

- **There are different kinds of healing, as we will see.** We often look *only* at "instant" healing as a valid form of the kingdom's in-breaking. But, we'll see that *choosing* to walk a pattern of health and wholeness is a valid form of healing as well- and was used by the Apostle Paul and even Jesus. In fact, Jesus commissioned His disciples to take this form of healing to others.

- In other words, **we were created to walk in healing, to experience health, and to enjoy the physical world around us.**

- **Our health should incorporate each part of our person: body, soul, and spirit.** We're created for *total* wellness. So, we shouldn't just limit health to our physical bodies, as we often do. Or, on the other extreme, limit health to our spirit.

C. Our goal = to outline a ___simple___ ___strategy___, three habits. These are routines you'll learn to do naturally.

1. The 3 habits are ___think___, ___touch___, and ___tell___.

- *Think* = believe the right things.

- *Touch* = reach out, anointing others as Jesus said you will do.[13]

---

[12] Dr. Henry Wright, *A More Excellent Way*, p12.

[13] Confession: I originally penned "Jesus said you *can* do." However, the thrust of Scripture is that healing is something we *will* do. We're already empowered to do it- we just need to awaken to that reality!

- *Tell* = declare the truth of the kingdom, praying and commanding healing to come.

Think, Touch, Tell

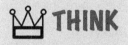 **Belief / faith**- deals with the important concepts of believing the right things about our Father, about healing, and about faith. This is, really, the starting point.

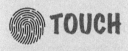 **Expression**- of sharing His heart with others, even without using words. In this section we will talk about the healing oils of the Bible.

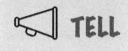 **Communication**- touching the entire person (body, soul, and spirit), carrying the presence and power of the kingdom with you, and focusing on what is right and pure...

2. All 3 habits are ___important___.

- *Think* = **the starting point.** Our actions reveal our beliefs. We either live based on truths or untruths. Without right thinking, the foundation is not present.

- *Touch* = **is a powerful way to overcome distance and hurt. Touch also has proven healing effects, too.** Perhaps this explains why Jesus touched the lepers when He healed them, even though the Bible clearly tell us that they were healed as soon as He spoke (Mark 1:41). *Without touching*, an element of intimacy is lower than it could be.

- *Tell* = **the Bible tells of the power of words.** We read that we overcome by the blood of the Lamb and the word of our testimonies (Revelation 12:11). And, "Life and death are in the power of the tongue" (Proverbs 18:21). "Faith comes by hearing," also, so you're generating faith and hope when you declare the truth (Romans 10:17). *Without telling*, people don't hear the revelation they need in the moment.

3. The 3 habits are __specific actions__ we'll teach. Each of the 3 habits is important for carrying __healing__ & __wholeness__ with you.

- Oddly enough, **these habits work in any relational context.** Lay hands on your children. On your spouse. On people who come to you for ministry.

- **These are routines you'll learn to do naturally-** as effortlessly as you reach for a cup of coffee in the morning, check your email / Facebook, or look in your rearview mirror when driving

- **Notice the graphics below and on the following page- and how these concepts fit together throughout the book.**

All 3 Are Important

♛ *-THINK* + TOUCH + TELL = LACKS STABILITY

☌ + THINK *-TOUCH* + TELL = LACKS INTIMACY

📢 + THINK + TOUCH − *TELL* = LACKS EXPRESSION

All Three Are Important!

Observation: Note that all three habits are important. Without telling, people don't hear the revelation they need in the moment. The expression of the heart of the Father is absent. Without touching, an element of intimacy is gone. And, without thinking, the foundation is not present. All three are important.

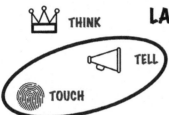

LACKS FOUNDATION

We are told to be transformed by the renewing of the mind (Romans 12:1-2). And, that "as a man thinks, so is he..." (Proverbs 23:7).

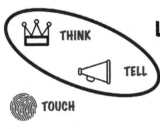

LACKS INTIMACY

In every instance, Jesus touched the lepers and those needing intimacy the most. He also sent His disciples to lay hands on the sick... knowing a physical touch is what many people need.

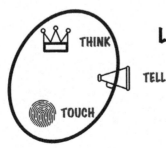

LACKS EXPRESSION

"Faith comes by hearing..." (Romans 10:17). And, we read, "How will they know unless someone tells them?" (Romans 10:14-15).

THE 3 HABITS

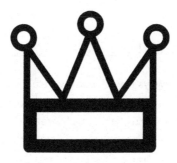

2. Habit 1 = Think

THINK RIGHT ABOUT WHO GOD IS
THINK RIGHT ABOUT FAITH
THINK RIGHT ABOUT HEALING

"Be transformed... by the renewing of your mind..." (Romans 12:1-2).

"Beloved, I pray that you may prosper in all things and be in health, just as your soul prospers" (3 John 2).

"For as he thinks in his heart, so is he" (Proverbs 23:7).

"Who forgives all your iniquities, Who heals all your diseases" (Psalm 103:3).

A. Think right about __who__ __God__ __is__.

- **Our actions always reveal what we truly believe.** In other words, our actions are simply the fruit of thoughts and belief structures. If we believe God is "for us," then, we'll feel and act differently towards Him than if we feel think He's against us. And, if we believe our Heavenly Father is *pro*-healing, we'll minister and live differently than we will if we feel He deliberately withholds healing- or even causes illness.

- **The starting point for anything in life is, really, understanding who God is.** By understating His nature, we get a better grasp of who we are and our ultimate destiny.

1. Jesus reveals __the__ __Father__.

- **Jesus told His disciples that He came to reveal the Father (14:9f.).** This concept appears repeatedly throughout the New Testament. We read:

    - *He is the image of the invisible God* (Colossians 1:15). If you want to see what God looks like, look at Jesus and you will see a perfect representation.

    - *He is the perfect imprint, the exact replication of God* (Hebrews 1:3). Jesus perfectly reveals the Father's glory.

- John 5:19 tells us when Jesus was walking on the earth that He *only* did what He saw the Father doing. This, according to Jesus, is why He did everything He did. Because of this, **we**

> WE KNOW WHAT THE FATHER IS LIKE BECAUSE WE SEE WHAT JESUS IS LIKE...

see the heart of the Father in every instance of Jesus ministering throughout the Gospels.

- Practically speaking, this means that **when you see Jesus doing something you actually see the Father doing that very same thing.**

  - Jesus preached grace and freedom to the woman caught in adultery- because *that's what He saw the Father doing* (John 8:3f.).

  - Jesus *touched* the leper rather than simply healing Him with a word- because *that's what He saw the Father doing* (Mark 1:41).[14]

  - Jesus ate with the tax collectors and sinners- because *that's what He saw the Father doing* (see Mark 2:15).

- **Notably, there are a few things *we do not see* Jesus doing-meaning that we do not see the Father doing them, either.**

  - *Condemning people-* we *never* see an instance of it.

  - *Causing illness-* we never see this, either, even though expressions like, "God gave me _____" (insert disease) or "God chose me for _____" (insert the ailment) are popular. Others say things like, "God gave me _____ to humble me / teach me a lesson, etc." But, we never see this in the life of Jesus.

2. Jesus Himself tells us _plainly_ what this all _means_.

- John 12:45 records Jesus saying plainly, **"If anyone has seen Me then they have seen the One who sent Me."**

---

[14] This is amazing, particularly when you realize that the leper was healed (according to Mark) as soon as Jesus spoke: "As soon as He had spoken, immediately the leprosy left him, and he was cleansed" (1:42). We see plenty of miracles in Jesus' ministry that He completed simply "with a word."

- And, 2 Corinthians 4:4 tells us that **Jesus is the image and likeness of God.**

- Therefore, **we know what the Father is like because we see what Jesus is like.** One pastor writes, "Jesus came to demonstrate who the Father is and what He is like, and He does so through His words and His actions. To gain a true picture of Father's feelings toward His children, it is best to turn to the One whose purpose it was to show us the Father. Jesus spent three years in ministry, demonstrating His Father's heart of compassion as He forgave sinners, healed the sick, and raised the dead."[15]

"

JESUS CAME TO DEMONSTRATE WHO THE FATHER IS AND WHAT HE IS LIKE, AND HE DOES SO THROUGH HIS WORDS & HIS ACTIONS...

— *Jack Frost, Experiencing Father's Embrace*

"

- **It's odd that the disciples missed this fundamental concept-** *just like we often do.*

  - "Even after all that time, Philip, one of Jesus' closest followers, echoed a sentiment that many Christians would still say, 'Show us the Father, and it is enough for us...'"[16]

  - Jesus then gave him the revelation of John 14:9-10: "He who has seen Me has seen the Father... the Father in Me does those works..."

---

[15] Jack Frost, *Experiencing Father's Embrace,* Kindle location 804.

[16] Jack Frost, *Experiencing Father's Embrace,* Kindle location 804.

- **Again, if you know what One is like, you know what the Other is like!**

  - If you've seen Jesus, *you've seen the Father.*

  - If you've heard the voice of Jesus, *you've heard the voice of the Father.*

  - If you know of something Jesus has done, *you also know of something amazing the Father has done.*

❝

ALL TOO OFTEN, MANY OF GOD'S CHILDREN MISTAKINGLY ASSUME THAT THEIR AFFLICTIONS ARE EVIDENCE OF GOD'S JUDGMENT ON THEM.

— *Jack Deere, Surprised by the Power of the Spirit*

❞

3. This is a __big__ __leap__ for a lot of people...

- **Old Testament vs. New Testament ideas / Law vs. Grace are prevalent.** We often believe that in the Old Testament we see what God is like, whereas the New Testament shows us what Jesus is like. We often believe that Jesus came to save us from God Himself![17]

---

[17] Do you disagree with this? Then ask yourself, "Who sends people to hell?" Then, "Who saves them from hell?" See what I mean? Most people will insist God sends people to hell, but Jesus saves them from hell.

- Yet all of the goodness we see in the New Testament actually comes from the Father![18]

- "Jesus came to demonstrate who the Father is and what He is like, and He does so through His words and His actions..."[19]

- "All too often, many of God's children mistakingly assume that their afflictions are evidence of God's judgment on them."[20]

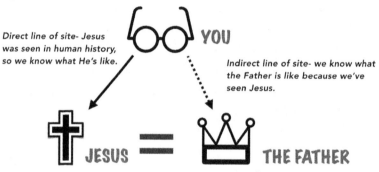

If You've Seen One, You've Seen Both

Direct line of site- Jesus was seen in human history, so we know what He's like.

YOU

Indirect line of site- we know what the Father is like because we've seen Jesus.

✝ JESUS = ♛ THE FATHER

4. Notice the ___radical___ ___difference___ in what Jesus did/didn't do.

---

[18] Still working through this theologically? The source of healing is the Father. It's made possible by Jesus' body and blood. Jesus is our Master and our Mentor- He tells us what we should do and shows us how to do it by His example. Remember, though, that He only did what He saw the Father doing (John 5:30, 8:38). Jesus' little brother, James even reminds us that "every good and perfect gift" still comes from the Father" (James 1:17). Yes, this is difficult to fit into a tidy theological box!

[19] Jack Frost, *Experiencing the Father's Embrace*, Kindle location 804.

[20] Jack Deere, *Surprised by the Power of the Spirit*, Kindle location 2357.

- **Jesus *never* caused sickness-** we never seen an instance of Him causing someone to be ill.

- The Bible tells us this: **Jesus went about healing *everyone*** (i.e., Matthew 4:23, Matthew 12:15).

- **Jesus actually used these healing miracles to confirm His identity- not call it into question** (see Luke 9:2, Luke 10:9).[21]

- **Jesus said that a kingdom divided against itself cannot stand** (Mark 3:24). In this passage, He asks, "Can Satan cast out Satan?" The implication is clearly... *no*, he cannot. Jesus brought this up in response to the religious leaders of the day who inferred that He had a demon- and that by the power of Satan He was casting out other demons.

> JESUS ACTUALLY USED THESE HEALING MIRACLES TO CONFIRM HIS IDENTITY- NOT CALL IT INTO QUESTION...

- Logically, we could apply this line of reasoning to healing. If God heals sickness today (we believe He does), then can we say the following: **If God causes sickness, He can't cast it out-** any more than Jesus could cast out demons if He had a demon. If sickness is of God- and from Him- wouldn't it be a schizophrenic house divided? **Why, also, would Jesus confirm His identity by pointing to His miracles?** He told John the Baptist, who questioned His identify, that the deaf hear, the lame walk, etc.[22] He told others that the healing were proof that the Kingdom was here.[23]

---

[21] This is according to Jesus' own witness about Himself. However, note that the religious legalists of the day *still* questioned Him. They argued that He was casting out demons (and presumably healing people) by the power of Satan (see Matthew 9:34, Matthew 12:24, Luke 11:15). Oddly enough, if you go to a Christian bookstore today, you'll find entire books where people spill a lot of ink making the same arguments!

[22] "Jesus answered and said to them, 'Go and tell John the things you have seen and heard: that the blind see, the lame walk, the lepers are cleansed, the deaf hear, the dead are raised, the poor have the gospel preached to them. And blessed is he who is not offended because of Me'" (see Luke 7:22-23 NKJV).

[23] Luke 9:2, 10:9

- As well, if we believe that God causes illness, would we not be fighting against His will (logically speaking) if we go to the doctor to try and heal what's happening with our bodies? Think about it. It's inconsistent- and it sets us in motion using natural means to fight the supernatural.[24]

Things from Jesus / Not from Jesus

THINGS JESUS DID	THINGS JESUS DIDN'T DO
HEALED EVERYONE	Cause illness / sickness / disease
FORGAVE	Condemn
REVEAL THE FATHER	Reveal... well... the other side

B. Think right about __faith__.

- Not only do we want to believe the right things about our Father, but **we also need to believe the right things about faith.**

- Often, **well-intended believers create a "work" out of faith-** and teach that you have to believe enough in order to "get" your healing.

---

[24] Henry Wright makes this point in *A More Excellent Way.* See p13 and p33 of his book. If God causes sickness to teach us a lesson, why would we try to get rid of it, instead of just learning the lesson? Wouldn't that be going against His will? Do you see what I mean? This line of argument doesn't really make sense once you step back and truly think about it.

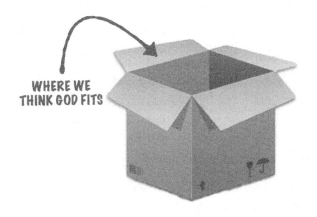

WHERE WE
THINK GOD FITS

1. I believe the Bible shows us that faith is not a
"__work__," a thing we must do to a certain measure in
order to ____earn____ our __healing__.

- **Many people argue that if you don't have enough faith God *cannot* heal.** In other words, these people wrongly assume we "handcuff" God's power by our lack of belief.

- When we look through the New
  Testament, though, we see something
  radically strange about the faith issue.
  Quite simply, **there is no formula on
  how much faith- or what kind of faith-
  is required for healing.** Sometimes,
  Jesus healed people who *didn't*

  > SOME PEOPLE
  > WRONGLY ASSUME
  > WE "HANDCUFF"
  > GOD'S POWER BY
  > OUR LACK OF BELIEF.

  believe; other times, He healed people who *totally* believed. He
  healed people who had *some* doubt mingled with *some* belief. Once,
  He even healed a man who didn't even know who He was!

2. When we see faith in the Bible, we notice that there is no " formula " or " box " we can fit everything into.

- **A "lack of faith" is not always a negative.** In the examples in the chart on the next page, the only person who made excuses was the lame man (John 5:1f.). The Bible says nothing negative about the other examples. In other words, this is a *neutral* issue- unless we are confronted with negativity. Do not immediately conclude that a "lack of faith" is a "deal killer" on the healing issue.

- **It was *not* a lack of faith that restrained Jesus from working miracles in his hometown** of Nazareth (see Mark 6:1f., Luke 4:16f.).

  > HONOR SEEMS TO BE MORE IMPORTANT THAN FAITH.

  - Rather, there was *no honor* present in His hometown (Mark 6:4, Luke 4:24). He was unable to do many miracles there (Mark 6:5). We assume He was unable to perform mighty works there because of the faith issue.

  - Notice what Mark writes, though: "A prophet is not without honor except in his hometown" (6:4). Then- "And He marveled because of their unbelief" (6:6). In other words, Mark seems to tell us, "In addition... He *also* was shocked because..." The issue that restrained Him was not a "faith issue" but an "honor issue."

- This honor issue also occurs in Luke 13:34-35, in which He says that He wants to gather the Lord's people together so they might experience His presence in a uniquely powerful way, but **they will not see Him until they honor those whom He sends.** (See also Matthew 10:40-42.)[25]

---

[25] This is a huge point that merits way more time and space!

- My point is this: **do not worry about someone's faith in what the Lord can do. If they are willing to receive ministry, *they will receive ministry*. If they are *not* willing to, they won't.** They must be able to accept it from you. Honor seems to be more important than faith.

- That said, **the only time I see someone healed according to the measure of their faith is when total faith is present** (see Matthew 9:29, for instance).[26] Jesus seems to say this almost as a commendation and recognition of extraordinary faith- not as an ingredient necessary for "earning" a healing (see the "total" faith examples in the chart which follows, in their specific contexts).

- **Jesus *never* criticized a "lack of faith" to people He was ministering healing**. Jesus never got mad at people for asking for a sign.[27] We often assume that He did- and some Christian traditions even suggest as much. However, note...

  - See Mark 9:14-29. A man has a demon-possessed son that convulses the boy, tosses him on the ground, and makes him foam at the mouth. As Jesus comes down the Mount of Transfiguration, He is met with this commotion. The disciples have been unable to cast out the demon.

  - Jesus issues a rebuke (9:23), but He clearly rebukes the disciples- *not the man in need* (9:29). Again, they already had authority to do this- and had successfully cast out demons in the past.

---

[26] Another instance is in Matthew 15:22f. Here, Jesus heals the Syro-Phoenician woman's daughter. She was clearly not part of the original mission, according to Jesus. He says He was sent to the lost sheep of Israel; she is a foreigner. Yet He is so moved by her great faith that He commends her and heals her daughter.

[27] Well, except for the Pharisees- but they were trying to trick Him. This goes back to the concept of honor.

A Lack of Faith is Not the Issue

FAITH ISSUE	SCRIPTURE	STORY
NO FAITH	John 5:1f.	Man at Bethsaida, lame for 38 years.
	Matthew 8:15	Simon Peter's mother-in-law, fever.
	Luke 13:12	Woman bent over for 18 years, cannot stand straight.
PARTIAL FAITH	Mark 9:24	"I believe, help my unbelief," cries father of the demon-possessed boy; disciples are chastised.
	Matthew 8:2	Leper approaches Jesus: "If you are willing..."
TOTAL FAITH	Matthew 9:18	Jairus tells Jesus to lay His hand on his sick daughter and she will live.
	Mark 7:24	Syro-Phonecian woman has her daughter healed of a demon. Her faith is commended.
	Luke 8:48	Woman with flow of blood: "If I touch His garment..."
	Matthew 9:29	Two blind men, "According to the faith."
OTHER'S FAITH	Mark 2:1f.	A paralytic is healed after his friends drop him through the roof and Jesus sees "their faith."
	Luke 7:1-9	Roman centurion, "Say the word..." (also, total faith).
WITH ACTION	Luke 17:14f.	The lepers, healed as they went
	Various scriptures	More about this in the notes below

- Again, Jesus criticized the disciples who were told to minister healing- and had previously been empowered to do it- and done it. He did *not* chastise those who *needed* ministry. The Father clearly has wavering faith, further adding emphasis to this point (see Mark 9:23-25).

- The takeaway? Do not rebuke people to whom you minister for their lack of faith. That is (somehow, even graciously) a burden that *we carry*- not a burden that they carry.[28]

> THE BIGGEST ISSUE- BIGGER THAN FAITH- SEEMS TO BE CONNECTED TO HONOR.

Honor > Faith

- **The biggest issue- bigger than faith- seems to be connected to *honor*, that is, to whether or not people are willing to receive ministry from you.**

- The chart on the previous page provides a few examples in each area. **Be sure to remember the final area on the chart- that sometimes the healing was backed by action.** However, remember that we simply take our thoughts captive to the "obedience of Christ" (2 Corinthians 10:5), and that through His actions (His life and His death), He accomplished everything required for us to be "one" with the Father and to experience our inheritance. We will come back to this point when we discuss walking a lifestyle of health and wellness.

---

[28] Do not feel like healing is out of bounds for you if your faith is wavering. The father in this story is the one who uttered the famous line, "I believe, help my unbelief!" He owned the fact that his faith wasn't whole, yet Jesus still healed his son!

- We don't work to earn something that Jesus has already provided; we do honor and steward His gift, however.

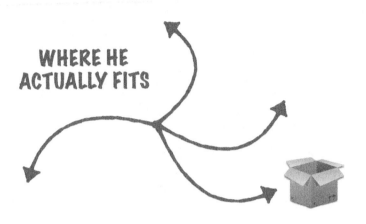

WHERE HE ACTUALLY FITS

C. Think right about ___healing___.

- We have discussed that there are core ideas we should believe about God (A.), and that we should "think right" about faith (B.). We should believe that:

  - *God is good* (A.), *and*

  - *Faith- or a lack of it- isn't an issue* (B.). It doesn't withhold the bounty of heaven. Nothing can separate us from His love (Romans 8:28f.).

- Now, we move to the third- and final- area where we need to "think right." **We must also "think right" about healing.**

So Far...

CORE AREA	THINK RIGHT...
GOD	God is good and loves His children. He doesn't harm them- He heals them.
FAITH	Faith is not a work we do to "earn" a healing. A lack of faith does not disqualify us for receiving healing. The bigger issue is honor- that is, if someone is willing to receive from us.
HEALING	

WE'LL UNPACK HEALING OVER THE NEXT FEW PAGES!

1. There are ___foundational___ ___concepts___ we should believe about healing.

- In this section we will see that **healing is broader than we often think.**

- **Healing can happen instantly- or "over time."** It can happen as what we might refer to as a *miracle*, or as a series of healthy choices and habits we choose to embrace.

- **Healing involves the total person- not just the physical body.** And, in fact, most healing will happens from the "inside out," as the spirit (the part of us that is one with God) and the soul (our mind, emotions, etc.) are addressed. When this happens, many times the physical symptoms simply disappear.[29]

2. **Three** different words refer to "**healing**" in the New Testament. Let's introduce **two** of them here.

- Understanding why different are words used is important as we begin a healing ministry- or even as we seek healing.

- Here are two of the Greek words (the New Testament was originally written in Greek and Aramaic) for *healing*.[30]

> UNDERSTANDING WHY THERE ARE DIFFERENT WORDS USED IS IMPORTANT AS WE SEEK HEALING.

  - *Iaomai-* means "miraculous" and "instantaneous" healing. This is how we most often envision Jesus healing, though this word only appears 30 times in the New Testament. (See examples in Matthew 8:13, Mark 5:29, Luke 8:47, John 12:40.)

  - *Therapeuo-* means "to serve, to attend to, or to wait upon menially" and "to heal gradually over time with care." This word appears 40 times in the Bible- a bit more than the instant cures we usually associate with miracles. (Matthew 4:23-24, Mark 1:34, Mark 6:13, Luke 5:15, Acts 5:16, Acts 8:7, Revelation 22:2.)

---

[29] We'll come back to these later in the book. For now, the "big two" internal issues seems to be these: 1) *forgiveness* and 2) *identity*. I've seen dozens of people healed simply by forgiving someone. We'll discuss some of the reasons perhaps why this happens when we discuss the limbic system later in the book. In addition, I've seen many people healed when they receive a revelation of their identity as a beloved child of a loving Heavenly Father.

[30] The discussion on the two Greek words comes from David Stewart's *Healing Oils of the Bible*. See p91.

3. I believe in- and have seen- _____ *iaomai* firsthand.

- My brother gouged an eye when he was younger. He was never supposed to be able to see. Today, **his eye is completely whole and has been for over 35 years. He's in his 40s and still doesn't even need glasses. That's** *iaomai*.

- My sister had a severe heart murmur when she was a small child. My parent's took her to a specialist in Houston who charted the arrhythmia. My Dad prayed and then took her back a few weeks later. The physician asked if they could use the new chart side-by-side in his classes with the old chart- one to show what a sick heart looked like on paper and the other to show what a perfect heart looked like. **They still use that chart 30-plus years later. Again, that's** *iaomai*.

- My uncle died twice at UAB. He came back. Twice. They didn't pump, aggressively resuscitate, or shock him. **The doctor walked to the waiting room both times and said, "Another miracle." That was over 15 years ago. Another** *iaomai*.

4. I also believe Jesus uses ___*therapeuo*___, that is, "___natural means___" over time to heal.

- Yes, I believe Jesus heals people in the moment. I also believe He can do things in other ways, too. Specifically, **I believe He can use natural means over time in the same way that He also uses medical professionals and miracles. It's** *all* **His healing, anyway.**

- **Now, we would say that** *all* **of Jesus' healings in the Bible were miracles.** None of us would make a list and say this one doesn't count, that one was normal, that one was something else… This wouldn't be up for debate!

- Yet, one of the words for "healing" that is used in the Gospels clearly shows us that Jesus didn't *always* heal immediately. Sometimes, He administered a series of instantaneous healings and other times He likely "taught people to be well."

- The word *therapeuo*, another word translated in English as "healing," appears significantly *more* times than *iaomai*, showing us there might actually be a slight emphasis here.

Two Words for Healing

	APPEARS	MEANING	HAPPENS
IAOMAI	30 times	Instantaneous healing	Spontaneously, in the moment
THERAPEUO	40 times	To serve, to attend to, or to wait upon menially- even by teaching them to be well	Intentionally, over time

5. ___**Both**___ types of healing happen in harmony with one another throughout ___**Jesus'**___ ministry.

- **Matthew 8 illustrates this healing spectrum.** Specifically, the stories in this chapter tell us "how" Jesus heals people. We will look at each of these instances and make a few more observations about healing in general. We will see both types of healing.

HABIT 1 = THINK

- **First, we see that Jesus absolutely heals instantly.** In one of His first miracles, Jesus goes to Peter's house.

  - There, we see Peter's mother-in-law is ill with a fever. Remarkably, Jesus touches her hand, the fever leaves her, and she serves them dinner (8:15). He heals her in a moment.[31]

  - This is an example of *iaomai*- just like my brother, my sister, and my uncle.

- **Second, we see that Jesus often teaches people to be well.** Word travels quickly about Peter's mother-in-law, and the townspeople began flocking to the house. Here's how it reads: "When evening came, many who were demon-possessed were brought to him, and He drove out the spirits with a word and healed all the sick" (Matthew 8:16, NIV).

  - Matthew 8:16 tells us that everyone in the town who is demon-possessed and sick is brought to Jesus. **He heals *all* of them**, according to the Bible (8:16).[32]

  - The phrase "with a word... healed all who were sick..." literally means, according to most Bible commentators that I've checked, "***He taught them to be well***" (8:16).

  - Want to guess what Greek word is used there in the New Testament? That's right, *therapeuo*, the second word for healing.

---

[31] She was probably deathly ill- this wasn't just a case of "higher-than-normal temperature." She was on her deathbed, I believe.

[32] Here's the tension today: Why aren't *all* people healed now? Clearly some are not healed. And, Psalm 103:3 tells us that our Father heals all of our diseases and forgives all of our sins. Both. To the same degree. Completely. Since our reality doesn't match what we see in the Bible, we've shifted to "disease management" rather than trying to understand why "all" aren't healed of "all" things. We're no longer looking for a cure- and prevention. This is odd because we don't question whether or not He forgives all sin!

iaomai

"

15 HE TOUCHED HER HAND AND THE FEVER LEFT HER, AND SHE GOT UP AND BEGAN TO WAIT ON HIM.

therapeuo

16 WHEN EVENING CAME, MANY WHO WERE DEMON-POSSESSED WERE BROUGHT TO HIM, AND HE DROVE OUT THE SPIRITS WITH A WORD AND HEALED ALL THE SICK.   *"He taught them to be well"*

"

6. We see both types of __*healing*__ in the Apostle Paul's ministry, too.

- Acts 28:7-9 tell us that he healed Chief Publius, who was on his death bed, sick with dysentery. **The Bible details that Paul *iaomai* him.** He instantly made him well.

- The remainder of the islanders gather to the hut, much in the same way that the crowds flocked to Jesus after He healed Peter's mother-in-law. Luke, a physician who is traveling with Paul, explains that **Paul then *therapeuo* the entire island.** That is, he taught them how to live well.

"

PAUL WENT IN TO SEE HIM AND, AFTER PRAYER, PLACED HIS HANDS ON HIM AND HEALED HIM.

iaomai

9 WHEN THIS HAD HAPPENED, THE REST OF THE SICK ON THE ISLAND CAME AND WERE CURED.

therapeuo

— *Acts 28:8-9 NIV*

"

7. Here's what it means that Jesus heals in ___two___ ___kinds___ of ways...

- **Sometimes, Jesus heals instantly. Other times, He teaches people how to be well.** Make note, sometimes Jesus touches us and we are *dramatically* changed in that moment. Other times, He imparts His wisdom to us so that we *can* be changed.[33]

What it means...

IAOMAI	THERAPEUO
HEAL LUNG CANCER	Teach ills of smoking
CURE DIABETES	Show how to eat better
HEAL STDs	Display beauty of true intimacy
HEAL PHYSICAL NUISANCES	Give directions on being alive!

---

[33] In John 5, we read the story of Jesus healing the man who sat paralyzed by the Pool of Bethesda. You probably know the story fairly well. He has been sick for 38 years. As such, he has gathered in a place where many sick people gather. They all believed that whoever jumped into the pool first, when the waters stirred, would be healed. He had likely seen people healed because he explained to Jesus that he had no one to push him in when the waters stir.

"Someone always jumps in ahead of me," he said, excusing his condition.

Jesus asked if he actually wanted to be well. The man offered excuses as to why he could not be. In spite of the man's reservations, Jesus healed the man. Notice that He didn't lay hands on the man; He simply commanded him to gather his things and walk! That is clearly *iaomai*.

Here's an oddity: **we later read that the man didn't even know it was Jesus that healed him,** because he's not certain who Jesus even is! The man begins walking and is instantly bombarded by the religious leaders. They chide him for carrying his mat on the Sabbath. A bit later, Jesus runs into the man (who, again, doesn't even know who Jesus is), telling him "go and sin no more, lest something worse happen to you" (worse than a 38-year illness!).

Here's where I think the concept of *therapeuo* comes into play here: The man received an instant healing, an *iaomai*. Now, though, he must walk in health and wholeness or he can become sick again. In other words, *therapeuo* and *iaomai* are not opposed to each other- they always complement and enhance.

- **Think about what this really means:**

  - Jesus can heal lung cancer- but *He can also teach us about the ills of smoking.*

  - He can cure diabetes- *He also shows us how to eat better.*

  - He can heal us of sexually transmitted diseases. *Also, He provides us with directions on how to live whole and healthy lives, as well as experience the joy of true intimacy.*

  - *He can heal us of the dozens of physical nuisances that we've grown to tolerate. Or, we can take His directions and experience what it really means to be alive!*

  - *He showed me the power of therapeuo beginning about two years ago!*[34]

Sometimes, Healing Comes as You Walk it Out

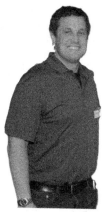

Unwellness- Many of the issues I faced were a direct result of the lifestyle I was living.

DOWN 50 POUNDS!

Wellness- I experienced two kinds of healing as I began living intentionally.

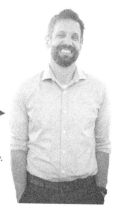

---

[34] This was an eye-opener for me. I had prayed for people before and seen instant miracles. I often wondered about the long-term results, though.

HABIT 1 = THINK

- **In the same way that I've seen *iaomai*, I've also experienced *therapeuo*.**

  - A few years ago, I was 50 pounds overweight.

  - Some of the symptoms I had included:

    - Low energy levels

    - I couldn't sleep well at night (Oddly enough, I could crash on the couch in the middle of the afternoon fine, however)

    - Digestive issues (blood in my stool, regularly; daily bouts with diarrhea)

    - Shortness of breath- even though I was exercising regularly

    - Creaking bones- and hardly able to walk- if I woke up in the middle of the night or when I woke up first thing in the morning

    - Constant need to urinate during the night (led to sleepless nights)

    - Inability to lose weight- regardless of my activity level

  - I made the decision to walk in wellness (*therapeuo*).

  - Some breakthroughs happened instantly.

    - I slept through the night immediately- and the snoring was gone.

    - My digestion issues all improved instantly- I believe it was an example of *iaomai*.

  - Other victories came as I continued walking in wellness, "walking out" my healing.

- Energy levels increased- and continued increasing

- I became stronger and stronger physically

- My thinking became much sharper

- Muscle and joint pain quickly diminished

- **You might be "healed as you go," too- just like I was *and* like the
ten lepers were who encountered Jesus** (see Luke 17:12-19).[35] Or
like Naaman the leper in the Old Testament, who was healed instantly
(2 Kings 5).[36] What's the difference? It's all His healing, anyway!
Remember the final category on the faith chart (page 33), that
sometimes action is necessary? To experience *therapeuo* there is
almost always an associated action!

8. We were designed to __choose life__, to __live well__.

- It's interesting that the leaves which bring healing are seen in the
Garden *before* sin entered the equation (Genesis 1:29) as well as *after*
the effects of sin are resolved (see Revelation 22:2).

    - *Why were there leaves for healing in the Garden of Eden,
    before sin entered the equation?*

---

[35] It has been my experience that people are often healed "gradually," as they walk in obedience. *They reap
more of the Kingdom harvest as they sow more into the principles of the Kingdom.* For instance, think
about the ten lepers that were healed as they obeyed Jesus, walking to show themselves to the priests (and
presumably to offer the required Levitical sacrifices) (Luke 17:14). In some instances, we see both of these
methods of healing working together: the power for the healing is given immediately, but people must
appropriate it by walking in the healing.

[36] Yes, on outward change could have happened instantly. God had the power to do this. But, I believe God
was more interested in using this situation to deal with Naaman's pride. Now, this doesn't mean that God
caused the leprosy to happen. However, Naaman was a better man afterwards because he was physically
well and he had dealt with the heart issue of pride. In the same way, I'm better and more disciplined, having
walked through the healing process rather than just having an instantaneous health change.

- *Why do we see leaves "for healing" in Heaven, where there's no more death & dying or sin?*[37] My thought: total health is our destiny. So, health now shows us a snapshot- even if a dim one- of our future.

- **It seems that walking in health and wholeness is a choice- in the same way that walking in intimacy is a choice.**

  - Adam & Eve chose to walk in relationship with their Heavenly Father. They were not "robots" without a free will.

  > WALKING IN HEALTH AND WHOLENESS IS A CHOICE- IN THE SAME WAY THAT WALKING IN INTIMACY IS A CHOICE.

  - Might they also have chosen to walk in health and wellness?

  - And aren't those choices- intimacy with our Father and walking in wellness- that we must make even now?

- **On the Cross, Jesus completed our intimacy *and* our healing**. That is, because of the Cross, our once-severed relationship with the Father is completely restored. In addition, we stand healed. The Bible tells us plainly: "By His stripes we are healed" (Isaiah 53:5).

  - Intimacy and healing are *past actions that have been completed* by Jesus.

  - We must choose to experience both, though. In other words, Jesus breaks the yoke of the original bondage, then *He teaches us how to walk in freedom*- in both areas.

---

[37] Genesis 1:29: ""I give you every seed-bearing plant on the face of the whole earth and every tree that has fruit with seed in it. They will be yours for [*oklah*]." Remember, *oklah* is food and medicines. These existed in the beginning before sin. I initially thought God was already making provision for sin. However, Revelation 22:2 shows us that the tree of life has an interesting function: "...On each side of the river stood the tree of life, bearing twelve crops of fruit, yielding its fruit every month. And the leaves of the tree are for *the healing of the nations*" (emphasis added). Notice, healing properties exist in Heaven- even though there is no sin there. The word used in Revelation 22:2 is *therapeuo*, by the way.

- Our encounter with Christ- and everything He provides- is not just a "one shot" encounter. Rather, **we are invited into an ongoing experience of the Kingdom.** "God said He not only forgives us all our iniquities, but He heals us of all our diseases."[38]

> BECAUSE OF THE CROSS, OUR ONCE-SEVERED RELATIONSHIP WITH THE FATHER IS COMPLETELY RESTORED. IN ADDITION, WE STAND HEALED.

- **Choosing wellness / *therapeuo* is your destiny (Revelation 22:2).**

Past Completed, Now Walk the Experience

	JESUS DID...	NOW, WE...
INTIMACY	Forgave sin, restored intimacy	Walk in the freedom of a relationship of grace
HEALTH	Healed, restored the body	Walk in health and wholeness

9. A 3rd word for healing, __SOZO__, shows us how comprehensive salvation- __total__ __healing__- truly is.

- **This word *sozo* is often translated as "saved" in the New Testament.** For instance, the Philippian jailer asks Paul, "What must I do to be saved / *sozo*?!" in Acts 16:31.

---

[38] Henry Wright, *A More Excellent Way*, p1.

- The word *sozo* means far more than "saved," however, and literally encompasses everything Jesus came to do.[39] The Word appears 101 times in the New Testament![40]

10. A series of miracles in Luke 7-8 shows us how broad *sozo* really is; these stories show us the __scope__ of salvation and the __depth__ of healing that is available even __today__.

- A woman of the street anoints Jesus' feet with her tears (Luke 7:36f.). He responds that her faith has sozo her (Luke 7:50). Clearly, **He has forgiven her sin.**

- Jesus rescues the disciples from a storm at sea (see Luke 8:24f.). Matthew, who was on the boat, records them as crying out to Him, "*Sozo* us!" (translated "Save us!") (see Matthew 8:25). **They obviously speak of their physical safety- *not* the forgiveness of sins**, even though the word is translated the same ("save").

> SOZO MEANS FAR MORE THAN "SAVED," HOWEVER, AND ENCOMPASSES EVERYTHING JESUS CAME TO DO.

---

[39] The name Jesus, Yeshua, actually means "salvation." He came to save people. He came to save people in a far greater way than we may have thought, however. It's important to note that Jesus came to offer a complete salvation, a salvation that affects the entire person. At the beginning of the Gospel of Matthew, we read that Mary should name her child Jesus. His name actually means "salvation, deliverance." The angel told her, "You shall call His name Jesus, for He will sozo His people from their sins" (Matthew 1:21). Throughout the story of His life on earth, we see that Jesus is consistently willing to sozo people (i.e., see Matthew 8:2). We never see Him denying anyone healing or deliverance. And, he's been far more successful at His work than we've often been taught!

[40] Source: http://www.biblestudytools.com/lexicons/greek/nas/sozo.html, accessed 05/16/2016.

- The demoniac, named Legion, approaches Jesus in Luke 8:26f. He is made *sozo* in Luke 8:36, and is found sitting in his right mind- even though he had been unclothed, tormenting himself in the tombs of the area. Obviously, **we see spiritual freedom / demonic deliverance.**

- Jesus raises Jairus' daughter from the dead (see Luke 8:40-42,49-56). Luke describes this as *sozo* (8:50), **the word he uses to denote raising the dead.**

- A woman with a flow of blood interrupted Jesus and Jairus' conversation in Luke 8:43f., when she reached out at touched Him, causing Jesus to feel power surge from Him. He declares that her faith has made her *sozo* (Luke 7:47). Here, **sozo refers to physical healing, meaning this is the third word we've seen for healing, marking it alongside *iaomai* (instantaneous healing) and *therapeuo* (healing, over time).**[41]

Total Healing

SOZO IS...	REFERENCE	WHAT HAPPENS?
FORGIVENESS	Luke 7:50	The woman of the street who fell at Jesus' feet
PHYSICAL PROTECTION	Luke 8:24 Matthew 8:25	The disciples, about to die in a storm at sea
DEMONIC DELIVERANCE	Luke 8:36	Legion is freed from hundreds of demons
RAISING THE DEAD	Luke 8:50	Jairus' daughter is brought back to life
PHYSICAL HEALING	Luke 7:47	The woman with the flow of blood is healed

[41] This seems to be an example of both *sozo* and *iaomai*, in my opinion.

11. Sozo is not only the __forgiveness__ of sins- it is the total reign of Jesus over all of life. It is the absolute __restoration__ and __reconciliation__ of all things.

Putting All 3 Healing Words Together

	APPEARS	MEANING	HAPPENS
IAOMAI	30 times	Instantaneous healing	Spontaneously, in the moment
THERAPEUO	40 times	To serve, to attend to, or to wait upon menially- even by teaching them to be well	Intentionally, over time
SOZO	101 times	Total salvation, over every area of life	Nothing is outside the scope & reign of Christ- forgiveness, physical protection / safety, spiritual deliverance, raising the dead, and physical healing are all possible

- **There is no area that is outside the scope of the Kingdom** (see Colossians 1:20). Jesus has been far more successful than you may have thought!

- **Many people have had an encounter with the "Gospel of the forgiveness of sin," which is in itself a beautiful message.** These people have prayed a prayer. They may have even walked an aisle. They believe in Jesus.

- **But Jesus told the Church to announce more, to walk in more.** To show the world- and to offer the world- a fuller way of life. To show a complete picture of God's goodness. To show what *sozo* means. You are invited into a total experience of the Kingdom right now!

> JESUS HAS BEEN FAR MORE SUCCESSFUL THAN YOU MAY HAVE THOUGHT!

12. The Church is called to preach the Gospel of the Kingdom, which we now see is broader than the __forgiveness of sins__ alone.

- **Jesus commanded His disciples-** *and empowered them-* **to preach the Gospel of the Kingdom when He sent them out. And, He told them to heal as they did** (Luke 9:2, for example).[42]

- **Notice the "kind" of healing He sends them to demonstrate and teach:**

  - When Jesus sends out the 70, He says: "Heal the sick there, and say to them, 'The Kingdom of God has come near...'" (Luke 10:9). The word He uses is *therapeuo*. They weren't just to instantly heal people (which we know they did from other places throughout the New Testament). They were told to teach a Kingdom way of life.

---

[42] They had to receive the healing, first- and then take it to others.

- Notably, this is the same way He sent the 12 in Luke 9:1-2. He "gave them power and authority over all demons, and to cure diseases." These two actions- *physical healing and spiritual deliverance*- were part of the complete salvation / *sozo* we just saw. Notably, "He sent them to preach the Kingdom... and to *therapeuo* the sick" at the same time" (NKJV). Instant healing and "healing over time" aren't at odds.

- We see this same dynamic happening in other Gospels. Matthew writes that Jesus told them, "Heal the sick, cleanse the lepers, raise the dead, cast out demons..." (Matthew 10:8 NKJV). Matthew says that Jesus said to *therapeuo* the sick... even while raising the dead and spiritually freeing the oppressed. Instant healing (*iaomai*) and healing over time (*therapeuo*) are present.

Walking in Health / Walking in Freedom

	HEALTH	SIN
IAOMAI **INSTANT**	We have been made whole	We have been forgiven
THERAPEUO **ONGOING**	We will walk in wholeness	We will walk in freedom from sin

Notice there are "instant" and "ongoing" aspects to both of the issues the Father resolves for us per Psalm 103:3. He forgives ALL sin; He heals ALL disease. Regarding sin, we are instantly forgiven- and we continue walking the experience of that intimacy. It effects every relationship we have. The same is true with our healing and our health!

13. We must decide what the practical application is for each of us...

- Where have we short-changed the true scope of salvation (read: *sozo*)? Are there areas we are wrongly believing are off limits- our "out of reach"- for God?

- Do we really believe that He still instantly heals (*iaomai*), that the Kingdom is among us and can manifest itself at any moment?

- What about *therapeuo*, about choosing to be well? And being confident to lead here?

    - How much of our unwellness is linked to our own actions? How many issues are caused by our actions? This could be our diet, our habits, environmental issues, toxic products we use, etc.

    - Did you know that physicians are now linking chronic illness- even major conditions like cancer- more with lifestyle choices than heredity or any other factors![43]

    - Scientists suggest that most physical ailments are caused by one of two issues:[44]

        - *Toxins entering the body* (that is, things that *should not* be there)

        - *Deficiencies of the body* (things that *should* be there are missing)

---

[43] "Lifestyle factors are involved in most cancers, with controllable factors estimated to be as high as 80 to 90 percent of all causes" (see https://pubs.ext.vt.edu/348/348-141/348-141.html, accessed 05/10/2016). And, "Only 5–10% of all cancer cases can be attributed to genetic defects, whereas the remaining 90–95% have their roots in the environment and lifestyle. The lifestyle factors include cigarette smoking, diet... sun exposure, environmental pollutants, infections, stress, obesity, and physical inactivity" (from http://www.ncbi.nlm.nih.gov/pmc/articles/PMC2515569/, also accessed on 05/10/2016).

[44] The following chart is adapted from my friend Jim Bob Haggerton. The first time I saw him use his version of this was in Florence, Alabama, at an event where he was speaking.

Two Causes of All Dis-ease

	1. TOXICITY	2. DEFICIENCY
THIS MEANS	My body comes in contact with things that it does not need, things which are harmful to it	My body is not receiving some of the things it does need, things which would benefit it
EXAMPLES INCLUDE	Sugar, artificial sweeteners, cigarette smoke, high fructose corn syrup, gluten, etc. (note: stress is a factor here, too!)	Dehydration, lack of sleep / rest, calcium deficiency, exercise / movement
SOLUTION INCLUDES	Purity- eliminating toxins whenever possible	Supplement- flooding my body with nutrients and other things that boost my wellness

- Have we embraced the idea that walking in *therapeuo* is really a spiritual issue?

- *Therapeuo* is an area where most people can *instantly* take control of their lives. Again, the Bible teaches both types of healing.[45]

- In embracing *therapeuo* and *iamoai*, you open yourself to a world of possibilities. **You have an amazing destiny, and incredible mark to make on this world. You cannot make your mark unless you are physically well.**

---

[45] Jesus healed everyone (Matthew 8:16). He said we would do greater works than He did (John 14:12). Can we not heal everyone, then?

- Bill Johnson writes, "None of us would say that He died for our sins but still intends that I should be bound by sin habits. Neither did He pay for my healing and deliverance so I could continue in torment and disease. **His provision for such things is not figurative. It is actual.**"[46] Think about how this applies to your wellness- and to the wellness of those to whom you will minister.

- By the way, *therapeuo* **is your destiny (Revelation 22:2). Enjoy the presence of your future now!**

> YOU CANNOT MAKE YOUR MARK UNLESS YOU ARE PHYSICALLY WELL.

---

[46] Bill Johnson, *Face to Face with Jesus*.

Walking in Therapeuo

Toxins & deficiencies I come in contact with each day- in my environment, etc. Much of this is out of my control.

Things I can control.

This is where you should focus

Notes: There are things you cannot control You cannot control the toxins you encounter in the workplace. Or the city in which you live. You CAN control the foods you eat, the movement you do (read: exercise), the many of the choices you make everyday which effect your health.

Where Do You Stand?

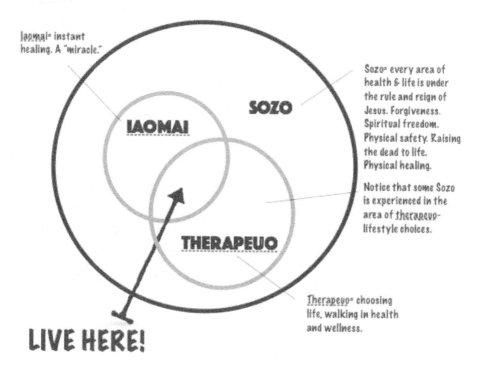

Iaomai= instant healing. A "miracle."

IAOMAI

SOZO

THERAPEUO

Sozo= every area of health & life is under the rule and reign of Jesus. Forgiveness. Spiritual freedom. Physical safety. Raising the dead to life. Physical healing.

Notice that some Sozo is experienced in the area of therapeuo-lifestyle choices.

Therapeuo= choosing life, walking in health and wellness.

LIVE HERE!

We can choose to live outside of the realm of the miraculous (outside iaomai) and stay only in healthy lifestyle choices (therapeuo). Or we can avoid both. The best place to live acknowledges God's hand in each- and recognizes every good thing of the Kingdom (sozo) can come in either form. Often, each type of healing works together!

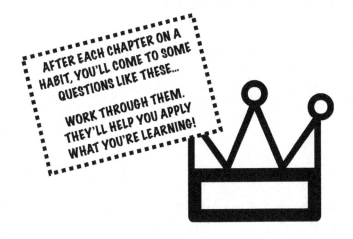

AFTER EACH CHAPTER ON A HABIT, YOU'LL COME TO SOME QUESTIONS LIKE THESE...

WORK THROUGH THEM. THEY'LL HELP YOU APPLY WHAT YOU'RE LEARNING!

Apply Habit 1 & Think

THINK RIGHT ABOUT WHO GOD IS
THINK RIGHT ABOUT FAITH
THINK RIGHT ABOUT HEALING

☐ Our actions always reveal what we truly believe. In other words, our actions are simply the fruit of thoughts and belief structures. If we believe God is "for us," then, we'll feel and act differently towards Him than if we feel think He's against us. We may say we believe one thing about God, but our actions will reveal what we really believe. That said, what do you believe about who God is, about faith, and about healing? How have you seen this manifest in your daily habits?

APPLY HABIT 1 & THINK

☐ Does God cause illness? If He does, then does it seem strange that we would try to cure it? If He doesn't, if He is the author of health and life, how do we get onboard with His plan for life and vitality?

☐ Here's the tension today: Why aren't *all* people healed now? Clearly some are not healed. And, Psalm 103:3 tells us that our Father heals *all* of our diseases and forgives *all* of our sins. Both. To the same degree. *Completely.* Since our reality doesn't match what we see in the Bible, we've shifted to "disease management" rather than trying to understand why "all" aren't healed of "all" things. We're no longer looking for a cure- and prevention. This is odd because we don't question whether or not He forgives all sin!

☐ Paul tells us that people in the Church at Corinth weren't healed because they were taking communion (read: celebrating the death of Jesus) without discerning His Body). Some Bible scholars believe that the blood makes forgiveness possible (without the shedding of blood there is no remission so sin, per Hebrews 9:22), and that the body makes healing possible (see Isaiah 53:5). We accept that our sins are forgiven (the blood), but we forget our bodies are healed as well (the body). One pastor writes, "We have eliminated one-half of the provision…"[47] What do you think?

---

[47] Henry Wright, *A More Excellent Way*, p21.

☐ What do you think it shows us that the word *therapeuo* is used more often in the Bible than the word *iaomai*?

Is There an Emphasis?

	APPEARS	MEANING	HAPPENS
IAOMAI	30 times	Instantaneous healing	Spontaneously, in the moment
THERAPEUO	40 times	To serve, to attend to, or to wait upon menially- even by teaching them to be well	Intentionally, over time

☐ Winning the lottery means nothing if you don't know how to manage the money. Most winners are broke within just a few months of winning. Many pro athletes find themselves in the same predicament. Can miracles (*iaomai*) work the same way? Without the ability- or choice- to walk in wellness and steward your healing, will it really work? In other words, is it accurate to assume that breakthroughs are important, but persistent is equally valuable?

APPLY HABIT 1 & THINK

☐ Notice the "faith chart" in this chapter. The final category says that faith is sometimes "backed by action"- and that is when some healing comes. I believe *therapeuo* is almost always the result of action, because it is a lifestyle, a series of steps we make every day. What do you think?

☐ What would it mean to truly be healed? How different would you be? Jesus asked the blind man and the lame man what they wanted Him to do for each of them. How might their identity have been wrapped in their condition? How might yours be? Once, when called for a blind man to come to him, the man "threw off his garment" (see Mark 10:50). In the ancient world, blind people wore garments to denote their identity- so this man was clearly shedding the old persona as he walked to Christ. What would you throw off?

☐ Intimacy and healing are both actions which were completed by Christ on the Cross. Now, we have the opportunity to choose both as an ongoing experience of the Kingdom. In what ways do each of these (forgiveness / intimacy and health / wellness) have both instant (*iaomai*) and ongoing (*therapeuo*) aspects?

Choosing Both- as a Way of Life

	JESUS...	NOW, WE...
INTIMACY	Forgave sin, restored intimacy	Walk in the freedom of a relationship of grace
HEALTH	Healed, restored the body	Walked in health and wholeness

You Were Created For...

Intimacy
WALK IN THE FREEDOM
OF A RELATIONSHIP
OF GRACE

& Health
WALK IN HEALTH
AND WHOLENESS

APPLY HABIT 1 & THINK

☐ I began this chapter stating there are things we see Jesus doing, as well as things we never see Him doing. Create your list of things you see / don't see.

THING JESUS DID	THINGS JESUS DIDN'T DO

JESUS HAS BEEN FAR MORE SUCCESSFUL THAN YOU MAY HAVE THOUGHT!

3. Habit 2 = Touch

ESSENTIAL OILS IN THE BIBLE
ESSENTIAL OILS EXPLAINED
ESSENTIAL OILS MOVE YOU HIGHER, FASTER

*"And these signs will follow those who believe: In My name they will cast out demons; they will speak with new tongues; they will take up serpents; and if they drink anything deadly, it will by no means hurt them; **they will lay hands on the sick, and they will recover**" (Mark 16:17-18 NKJV).*

*"Is anyone among you sick? Let him call for the elders of the church, and let them pray over him, **anointing him with oil in the name of the Lord.** And the prayer of faith will save the sick, and the Lord will raise him up" (James 5:14-15 NKJV).*

"So they went out and preached that people should repent. And they cast out many demons, and anointed with oil many who were sick, and healed them" (Mark 6:12-13 NKJV).

A. We see ___essential___ ___oils___ throughout the Scripture.

- **Essential oils are an integral part of the healing ministry in the Scriptures.** We have as much detail about the oils as we do about baptism, the Lord's Supper, and some other fundamental practices in our faith. Yet, in our Western culture of allopathic care, we often miss this one![48]

1. The tree of life and the trees in the Garden of Eden were full of the __power to heal__.

- See the Intro, the explanation of *oklah* as "foods and medicines." **The first time God gave plants to man, He was giving food *and* healing.**[49]

- The "law of first mention" is a Bible study principle that means that anytime we see something in Scripture, we should **look to the first time it appears to see how we**

> ESSENTIAL OILS ARE AN INTEGRAL PART OF THE HEALING MINISTRY IN THE SCRIPTURES.

---

[48] Allopathic care = western medicine. It consists primarily of disease treatment rather than prevention. It leans heavily on medicines, pharmaceuticals, interventions, etc., as opposed to lifestyle changes and natural approaches.

[49] See the introduction to this book, point B.

should interpret it. This, should effect how we view the world around us.

- **Plants aren't just food; they are healing.**

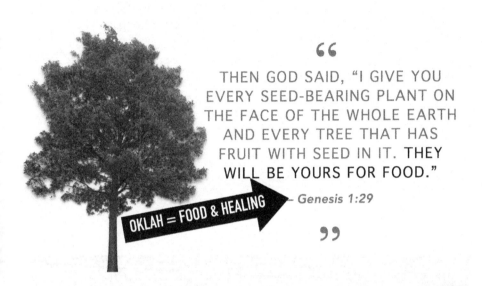

66

THEN GOD SAID, "I GIVE YOU EVERY SEED-BEARING PLANT ON THE FACE OF THE WHOLE EARTH AND EVERY TREE THAT HAS FRUIT WITH SEED IN IT. **THEY WILL BE YOURS FOR FOOD."**

— Genesis 1:29

99

OKLAH = FOOD & HEALING

2. The ___*healing*___ ___*properties*___ of plants have been used throughout history. Many cultures have been using them since Creation. They are not an isolated phenomena.

- "Ancient texts and historical and archaeological evidence- including Egyptian hieroglyphics, Chinese manuscripts, Greek physicians' records, and Biblical references- suggest that **essential oils have been an integral part of health and wellness for centuries.**"[50]

---

[50] Scott Johnson, *Surviving When Modern Medicine Fails*, p8.

> "
>
> ANCIENT TEXTS AND HISTORICAL AND
> ARCHAEOLOGICAL EVIDENCE- INCLUDING
> EGYPTIAN HIEROGLYPHICS, CHINESE
> MANUSCRIPTS, GREEK PHYSICIANS' RECORDS,
> AND BIBLICAL REFERENCES- SUGGEST THAT
> ESSENTIAL OILS HAVE BEEN AN INTEGRAL PART
> OF HEALTH AND WELLNESS FOR CENTURIES.
>
> — *Scott Johnson*
> *Surviving When Modern Medicine Fails*
>
> "

HIPPOCRATES, THE FAMOUS GREEK PHYSICIAN,
THE "FATHER OF MODERN MEDICINE," USED
ESSENTIAL OILS AS HIS MEDICINES

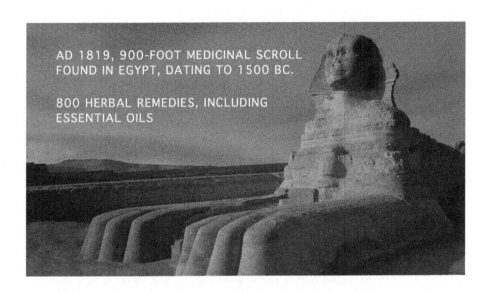

AD 1819, 900-FOOT MEDICINAL SCROLL FOUND IN EGYPT, DATING TO 1500 BC.

800 HERBAL REMEDIES, INCLUDING ESSENTIAL OILS

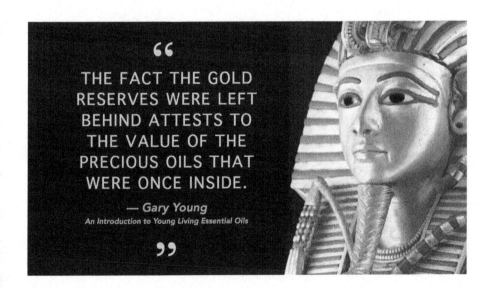

" THE FACT THE GOLD RESERVES WERE LEFT BEHIND ATTESTS TO THE VALUE OF THE PRECIOUS OILS THAT WERE ONCE INSIDE.
— Gary Young
An Introduction to Young Living Essential Oils
"

- Hippocrates, a famous Greek physician, used essential oils as his medicines.

- 1819, **a 900-foot long papyrus was found in Egypt, dating to 1500 BC. It is believed to be a "medicinal scroll,"** and contains over 800 herbal prescriptions and remedies as well as references to essential oils.[51]

- 1922, King Tut's tomb was discovered. The crew which explored the tomb found 50 alabaster jars (which would have held 7 liters of oil each, for a total of 350 liters total). Raiders had taken the oil but left the gold behind. **"The fact the gold reserves were left behind attests to the value of the precious oils that were once inside."**[52]

> PLANTS AREN'T JUST FOOD; THEY ARE HEALING.

- **"Kings would barter and buy land, gold, and slaves with their crudely extracted oils, because they were more valuable than gold."**[53]

3. From Egypt to the Tabernacle and through the Old Testament, __essential__ __oils__ prove __relevant__ to what God was doing.

- **There are 200 references to essential oils in the Old Testament alone.**[54]

---

[51] Gary Young, *An Introduction to Young Living Essential Oils*, p3.

[52] Gary Young, *An Introduction to Young Living Essential Oils*, p3.

[53] Gary Young, *An Introduction to Young Living Essential Oils*, p3.

[54] Review Dr. Stewart's book *Healing Oils of the Bible* for a detailed overview.

- One of the big focal points of the Old Testament is the Tabernacle.[55] **God gave specific instructions about the Tabernacle and even the oils used in it.** The Lord gave very specific instructions, also, about the building of the Tabernacle, the furniture and relics that were to be placed inside, and the adornment of the priests who would administer specific sacrifices.

The Old Testament

Essential oils appear 200x

Central to the Tabernacle

Priests anointed with a specific blend

- He was clear, too, that **those priests were to be anointed with a *specific* blend of essential oils which He relayed to Moses**:

    - "Take the finest spices: of liquid myrrh 500 shekels, and of sweet-smelling cinnamon half as much, that is, 250, and 250 of aromatic cane, and 500 of cassia, according to the shekel of the sanctuary, and a hin of olive oil. And you shall make of

---

[55] Particularly in the time of Moses, we see the prominence of essential oils. There are well over 200 references. The Egyptian connection makes sense when you remember that Moses was steeped in Egyptian tradition. He was a true "prince of Egypt" and raised as such, until he fled for his life after killing a fellow Egyptian in the fields.

these a sacred anointing oil blended as by the perfumer; it shall be a holy anointing oil" (Exodus 30:23-25, ESV).

- For mathematic purposes, 500 shekels is about one gallon.[56] In effect, Moses was blending the following:

  - Myrrh- 1 gallon (500 shekels)

  - Cinnamon- 1/2 gallon (250 shekels)

  - Calamus- 1/2 gallon (250 shekels)

  - Cassia- 1 gallon (500 shekels)

  - Olive oil- about 1 & 1/3 gallons ("a hin" is slightly larger)

- When complete, he had the equivalent of a *five gallon bucket* of anointing oil. If they didn't ration it when applying the anointing oil, it would *drench* the man being anointed.

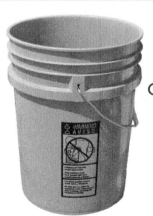

The Anointing Oil

MYRRH 1 gallon (500 shekels)

CINNAMON 1/2 gallon (250 shekels)

CALAMUS 1/2 gallon (250 shekels)

CASSIA 1 gallon (500 shekels)

OLIVE OIL 1 & 1/3 gallons (a hin)

---

[56] See *Essential Oils Pocket Reference*, pp6-7.

> 66
>
> BEHOLD, HOW GOOD AND PLEASANT IT WHEN BROTHERS DWELL IN UNITY!
>
> IT IS LIKE THE PRECIOUS OIL ON THE HEAD, RUNNING DOWN ON THE BEARD, ON THE BEARD OF AARON, RUNNING DOWN ON THE COLLAR OF HIS ROBES!
>
> IT IS LIKE THE DEW OF HERMON, WHICH FALLS ON THE MOUNTAINS OF ZION! FOR THERE THE LORD HAS COMMANDED THE BLESSING,
>
> LIFE FOREVERMORE.
>
> *— Psalm 133:1-3 (ESV)*
>
> 99

- Consider the passage above Psalm 133:1-3 (ESV).

- Notice that the oil flows down the robes as it falls off the priest's head, fills his beard, and hits the collar. **That's *a lot* of oil!**

- **Some people in the Tabernacle had the specific job of maintaining the oil.** They were known as "perfumers" (see 1 Chronicles 9:30, Nehemiah 3:8).

- **Other oils were used during Korah's rebellion** (see Numbers 16:30) and during the following day when others complained (see Numbers 16:49-50).

  > ESSENTIAL OILS ARE AN INTEGRAL PART OF THE HEALING MINISTRY IN THE SCRIPTURES.

- **We actually see essential oils before the time of Moses in the Bible** (still connected to Egypt, though). Consider this bit of irony from Joseph's story:

- He was sold by his brothers to a caravan of essential oil traders.[57] The Promised Land sat at a geographic crossroads in the Middle East, strategically creating an amazing location to conduct business. This is likely how Solomon expanded his empire.

- We know that the caravan was on the way through the Promised Land to Egypt with spices, balms, and myrrh (Genesis 37:25).

- One irony, of course, is that the brothers who sell Joseph must later appear before him to have their lives spared!

- Here's the greater irony: Jacob, their father, sends them back to their brother (not knowing that it is Joseph- he has not yet revealed himself to them!) with a gift of the exact same essentials oils they traded him for (Genesis 43:11)!

- We read that the incense of the Temple was of a sweet smell (see Exodus 30:25f.). Notably, it was common in those days for public areas to have essential oils diffusing throughout the building. The Romans cleansed public buildings with them (we will see that oils can purify things as well as people). In other words, **essential oils were in common use culturally.**[58]

"FRANKINCENSE IS GOOD FOR EVERYTHING FROM HEAD TO TOE."

- Ancient Egyptian Proverb

---

[57] See David Stewart's *Healing Oils of the Bible*, xviii.

[58] *Essential Oils Pocket Reference*, p5.

4. We even see ___*essential*___ ___*oils*___ in Jesus' life and ___*ministry*___.

- **Jesus' additional name, Christ- or *Christos*- means "anointed one."**[59] **When priests and kings were set into office, they were anointed with essential oils.**[60] And, they were put in place for a specific purpose. Of course, Jesus came to *save*, which we discussed earlier.[61]

- At His birth, **the magi brought Gold, Frankincense, and Myrrh. Notably, two of the three items are essential oils.** The ancients believed Frankincense had great healing properties- it was common for doctor and healers to carry both Frankincense and Myrrh with them.[62]

  - "Myrrh is still recognized for its ability to help with infections of the skin and throat and to rejuvenate tissue. Because of its effectiveness in preventing bacteria growth, myrrh was also used for embalming."[63]

> CHRIST- OR CHRISTOS- MEANS "ANOINTED ONE." WHEN PRIESTS AND KINGS WERE SET INTO OFFICE, THEY WERE ANOINTED WITH ESSENTIAL OILS.

---

[59] In Acts 10:38 we read: "...how God anointed Jesus of Nazareth with the Holy Spirit and with power, who went about doing good and healing all who were oppressed by the devil, for God was with Him" (NKJV).

[60] When was Jesus anointed? We read that He was anointed by a woman of the street multiple times- including at the beginning of His ministry and at the end, preparing Him for the Cross (see Luke 7:36f and Mark 14:3f.). These instances are at the homes of two different men, and they happen at two different times. Since these are from two of the "synoptic Gospels" we can presume they are following a similar timeline of Jesus' life. The two writers simply record two different events.

[61] See the discussion on the word *sozo* (chapter 2- Habit 1: Think, B., 9.).

[62] Consider what you would bring to a king if you could bring anything of great value?

[63] *Essential Oils Pocket Reference*, p5.

- Did Jesus use Myrrh with the lepers? Given the fact that many traveling healers in the day would have had both Frankincense and Myrrh with them at all times, it seems plausible to think so.

- Does this make the Bible stories less dramatic, less supernatural? *Not at all.* If anything, it makes the experience of these truths more accessible. Face it, sometimes *iaomai* seems out of reach; *therapeuo* is always at hand, however.[64]

- **When Jesus sent His disciples out, He sent them to heal-** *while laying their hands on people with oils.*

  - Mark 6:7-13 records perhaps the first instance of this: "And He called the twelve to Himself, and began to send them out two by two, and gave them power over unclean spirits... And they cast out many demons, *and anointed with oil* many who were sick, and healed them" (NKJV emphasis added).

  - Jesus' younger brother, James, gives the same instructions to early church leaders: "Is anyone among you sick? Let him call for the elders of the church, and let them pray over him, *anointing him with oil* in the name of the Lord" (James 5:14 emphasis mine).

- **It seems that the oils were legitimate, full strength oils- not symbolic oils.** Remember, when Jesus was anointed with Spikenard, the argument was related to the cost (see Mark 14:1-9, Matthew 26:1-13). The oil used to anoint Him was worth a year's wages of a common laborer. We will discuss the importance of the quality of the oils used

> FACE IT, SOMETIMES IAOMAI SEEMS OUT OF REACH; THERAPEUO IS ALWAYS AT HAND, HOWEVER.

---

[64] And, as we discussed earlier, even when a miracle comes, you maintain the healing by walking in *therapeuo.*

in a moment.

- **We known Jesus' body would have, historically speaking, been prepared for burial with oils, too.** Joseph of Arimathea and Nicodemus prepared Jesus' body for burial (John 19:39).[65] They needed a large quantity of essential oils do to this (about 100 liters- or 75-100 pounds). This would be worth about $150,000- $200,000 in today's retail environment, showing 1) their great wealth as well as 2) their great reverence for Jesus.

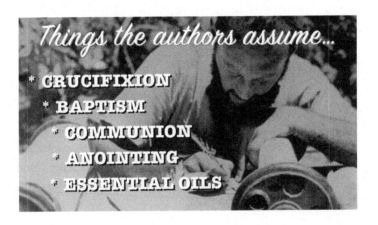

5. What's being assumed by the Gospel writers? A __lot__ about __several__ __important__ subjects.

- **The authors of the Bible simply assume we know some the basics of essential oils.** There are hundreds of references throughout the Bible meaning the authors must have assumed we would know what was being referenced. The truth is that their *immediate* audience did know!

---

[65] You may remember that Jacob was buried in Genesis 50:26. According to the embalming customs of the Egyptians who buried him, his body would have been treated with such oils also. See *Healing Oils of the Bible*, p140.

- This is simply how they wrote- there are *many* predominant ideas that the authors of the Bible never explain, simply assuming we'll know what they're talking about. For instance:

  > THERE ARE MANY PREDOMINANT IDEAS THAT THE AUTHORS OF THE BIBLE NEVER EXPLAIN, SIMPLY ASSUMING WE'LL KNOW WHAT THEY'RE TALKING ABOUT.

  - *Crucifixion*, the centerpiece of the New Testament- and the very act that most of the Old Testament points to- is never explained. Yet, it remains the focal point of the Bible and, really, human history.

  - *Baptism* is never explained- hence, much of the disagreement throughout Church history as to the proper way to baptize someone.

  - *Communion*- or the "Lord's Supper"- isn't really explained in any detail, either. In fact, the way they practice communion in the Bible seems radically different than how we do it. They seem to celebrate with an entire meal (see 1 Corinthians 11).

  - *Anointing* appears throughout the Bible. Strangely, we don't see many details on this, either. (Incidentally, the act *never* seems symbolic in Scripture; it appears that something actually happens in the moment of the anointing, as well.)[66]

  - Finally, *essential oils* appear in the Scripture hundreds of times.[67] Though someone living in Jesus' day would know what the authors meant when they referred to oils (or any of

---

[66] We've gotten so confused about this one that we've even changed the name to *ordination* in some church circles to just "start over" with a new concept.

[67] "The Bible contains 33 species and more than 500 references to essential oils and the aromatic plants from which they came" (Stewart, *Healing Oils of the Bible*, p7).

the other important concepts listed above- *crucifixion, baptism, communion, anointing*), we typically don't.

- **Some people may make the case that they didn't have doctors, then, so they relied more on natural means.**

    - It may be true that, partly. I think we actually rush to medical professionals today because of their easy access. If they weren't so accessible, we might take more responsibility for some of our health choices.

    - Oddly enough, "doctors" appears in the Bible *three* times (see Luke 2:46, Luke 5:17, and Acts 5:34).[68] In each instance, written by Luke (a physician, who would know what a *doctor* is), the reference is to "doctors of the law"- meaning *rabbis* or *teachers* as opposed to practitioners of healing.

    - Physicians were ordered to prepare Jacob's body for burial (Genesis 50:2). From this story, we learn that they were practitioners of essential oils. And, we see Luke repeatedly referring to the concept of *therapeuo*.[69] Perhaps there is a strong link here.

6. The __*healing*__ __*power*__ of touch... is both ancient and new.

    - A few pages ago we noted that Jesus touched the leper- even though He is able to (and does, throughout the New Testament) heal with just a word. **To a person who has experienced isolation, human touch is powerful.**

---

[68] *Healing Oils of the Bible*, p49.

[69] Remember, Luke (a doctor) is actually the most prolific author in the New Testament.

TOUCH

=ONE OF THE MOST POWERFUL HUMAN FORCES

- In fact, **modern science suggests human touch is one of the most powerful forces.**

  - "We come equipped with an ability to send and receive emotional signals solely [by touch]. In one experiment participants communicated eight distinct emotions- anger, fear, disgust, love, gratitude, sympathy, happiness, and sadness- with accuracy as high as 78 percent."[70]

  - "I have witnessed the power of healthy touch to heal, deliver, redeem, and restore people in mind, body, and spirit. Loving touch has the power to draw out the introverted autistic child, make an outcast teenager feel loved and accepted, or communicate safety to a battered woman. Healthy, loving touch reminds us of our God-given worth and identity."[71]

  - "According to neuroscientists, our brains are programmed for touch."[72] The study cited in this article actually shows that "touchier teams" (i.e, basketball, football) performed better than less touchier teams. Apparently, something is

---

[70] "The Power of Touch,," by Rick Chillot, *Psychology Today*, published March 11, 2015.

[71] "Have We Forgotten The Power of Touch?" by Nicole Watt, in *Christianity Today*, June 6, 2014.

[72] "Power of Touch a Transformative, Healing Force." See CBN News, CBN.com, September 8, 2014.

communicated in the high-fives, the shoulder taps, and the fist bumps that is actually quantifiable.

- **Perhaps it makes more sense, now, that laying on of hands is almost always mentioned with healing** (this happens in other instances, too, when something powerful is happening, such as the declaration of a new identity or destiny). In fact, the laying on of hands- *touch*- is mentioned in several powerful ways throughout Scripture. Touch is so important that it's not just limited to healing.

    1. *Healing-*

        - Mark 6:5 (Hands were laid on people- and they were healed.)

        - Mark 7:32 (People beg Jesus to lay hands on a man who is deaf and mute.)

        - Mark 16:17-18 (Jesus says His followers will lay hands on the sick.)

        - Luke 4:40 (Jesus laid hands on people who were brought to Him from throughout the village, even into the evening.)

    2. *Imparting spiritual gifts / supernatural power to do something-*

        - 1 Timothy 5:22 (Paul cautions Timothy not to lay hands on new leaders too soon; he actually imparts some power to them when he does.)

        - 1 Timothy 4:14 (Gifts are imparted by the elders to others stepping into ministry roles- would this be like an anointing? Did it involve oils?)

        - Deuteronomy 34:9 (Moses gives Joshua wisdom.)

    3. *Blessing people-* Mark 10:16 (Jesus laid His hands on the children and blessed them.)

4. *Imparting the Holy Spirit*- Acts 8:17 (Peter and John laid hands on the Samaritans and the Holy Spirit was imparted to them.)

- **Question: Were these instances of "laying on of hands" simply instances when people were touched by another? Or did they operate like times of an anointing (which we will discuss in a moment), instances where**

> DID THEY OPERATE LIKE TIMES OF AN ANOINTING... INSTANCES WHERE MORE THAN A SIMPLE TOUCH OCCURRED?

more **than a simple touch occurred?** Is James giving us details about laying on of hands (he includes oils) that would have been commonly practiced? We know that when kings and priests were anointed, oils were used. We also know that when Jesus sent the disciples to lay hands on the sick, He instructed them to use oils. Was this the common practice for each of the verses above? Is this what we would expect to see if we were present in those instances? For the answer, let's take a deeper look at essential oils and how they are used.

LAYING ON OF HANDS

* HEALING

* GIFTS / POWER

* BLESSING

* HOLY SPIRIT

B. Essential oils __explained__.

1. Essential oils aren't the same as the __other__ __oils__ in your home.

- **You probably already have several oils in your home.** You may have vegetable oil, peanut oil, or olive oil in your cupboard. These oils are great for cooking, for providing fuel for lanterns, etc., but the are "fatty oils" which will clog your pores if placed on your skin.

- **Household oils, however, have a different purpose that essential oils.**

2. Essential oils are __aromatic__, __volatile__ liquids. They are compounds found within shrubs, flowers, trees, roots, branches, and seeds (depending on the plant). The __life__ __source__- or __essence__- of the plant, they are usually extracted through steam distillation.

- **As the life source of the plant, they are to the plant what blood is to humans.**

- **They are unique to each plant, each having different characteristics.**

3. There are different "__grades__" (read: __qualities__) of essential oils. All oils are not created equal!

Quality Continuum- 3 Grades of Oils

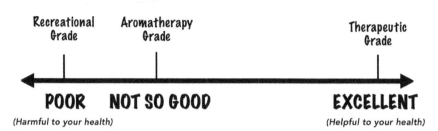

| Recreational Grade | Aromatherapy Grade | | Therapeutic Grade |

POOR **NOT SO GOOD** **EXCELLENT**

(Harmful to your health) *(Helpful to your health)*

Notes: Recreational Grade products are on one extreme- and are even harmful to you. Therapeutic Grade products are helpful- on the far other extreme. Notice that this is not an instance of "good, better, best." There are radical differences between the three grades.

Comparison of the 3 Grades of Oils

GRADE	CHARACTERISTIC	WHAT IT MEANS
RECREATIONAL GRADE OILS	Is basically a liquid with a synthetic smell added. These are for entertainment value- or symbolism- only.	They are actually harmful as they are toxic (which is why your body reacts to the smell, often).
AROMATHERAPY GRADE OILS	Have "fillers" that have been added to make them stretch and fill more bottles.	They simply do not work as well. If you use these, you may not actually get any benefit. This might lead you to think that "essential oils" don't work (when, really, you just used an inferior product).
THERAPEUTIC GRADE OILS	These are pure. If it doesn't grow, you don't get it.	Your body can make use of these, because they are natural and pure.

- One educator taught us that **"Everything that's labelled 'essential oil' is not necessarily the same."**[73] Some manufacturers "cut" oils and add fillers to stretch them; others add synthetic fragrances (such that the majority of the "oil" is simply a lab-created smell).

- **Here are three of the predominant grades of oils:** *recreational, aromatherapy, therapeutic.*

    1. *Recreational Grade*- is the lowest grade of oils (and other fragrances). Most of what is sold at Christian book stores falls in this category (or most stores, for that matter).

        - "Many companies have jumped onto the aromatic bandwagon solely for commercial reasons. They market products that are made solely for… *recreational fragrancing.*"[74]

        - Air fresheners, scented candles, car fresheners, and other items commonly found in big box retail stores are simply "smells" that have been artificially created.[75] They have no health benefits. In fact, studies are now showing that most of these lab-created synthetics are actually harmful for you.[76]

---

[73] See Young Living's *Core Vigor and Vitality*, p5.

[74] This quote comes from Daniel Penoel in Gary Young's *An Introduction to Young Living Essential Oils*, iii. Emphasis added. What are some examples of companies hopping on the bandwagon? Well, this past Christmas, Target, Walmart, and even Barnes & Noble began selling essential oils and diffusers. They weren't doing this for health reasons or they would have been in the market long ago. Rather, they were doing this to capitalize on current consumer spending trends. Recently, Barnes & Noble placed their remaining items on clearance. You won't be able to depend on them for a long-term health solution, because 1) the quality they provide is simply recreational in nature, as well as 2) you can't make repeat purchases.

[75] Think about it: scents like "cinnamon roll" and "birthday cake" do not appear in nature. To have these scents in a candle, they must be artificially created. They have detrimental effects because they tinker with the limbic system while introducing harmful chemicals into your body.

[76] For instance, see https://branchbasics.com/blog/2015/01/fragrance-is-the-new-secondhand-smoke/ (archived April 11, 2016).

- If you've ever reacted to the smell of a cleaning product or a cologne, your body is alerting you to a lab-created fragrance. *Nothing is wrong with you in that moment.* In fact, just the opposite. Your body is reacting, informing you that something isn't right. Your body can absorb- and utilize- natural products. However, it can't do anything with synthetics any more than it can digest and convert fast food into nutritional fuel.

- If you're using something (a candle, air freshener, spray, etc.) for a smell- or for symbolism- rather than an actual health benefit- you're probably using a "recreational grade" product. And, rather than having a health benefit, it probably has a health hindrance. Or, to refer to the chart we created earlier, it's not supplemental to your health; *it's toxic.* And, remember, sickness is caused by toxins (things in your body that shouldn't be there) and deficiencies (things missed which should be present).

2. **Aromatherapy Grade**- this grade is slightly better than recreational grade oils , as well as a bit cheaper than the final (and best) category, therapeutic grade. These oils have authentic elements to them, but are watered down with fillers.[77] The essential parts of the plant are stretched so the producer may fill more bottles. You can't ingest these oils- usually the bottle will actually warn you not to do so.

    - This name is tricky, because it actually sounds more important than it is to most people. In Great Britain, people take it for granted that an "aromatherapy

---

[77] Why would someone alter the oils? Here are a few obvious reasons: Your profit margin is higher if you can stretch the product. More people will buy a *cheaper* product, not realizing that quality matters (who wants to spend $10.00 on a single incense stick when they can buy *five* for $1.00?). Your shelf life is longer (food people have known this for years- hence, all the additives and preservatives).

grade" oil is an oil to be used for massage. The title denotes the oil has clearly been diluted with a carrier oil, stretching it to make it last longer. Since we are not as familiar with some of these terms in the United States, though, we often mistakingly thing that "aromatherapy" means high quality.

- Whole Foods sells aromatherapy grade oils; Walmart, Barnes & Noble, and Target sell recreational grade- by comparison.

3. **Therapeutic Grade**- this is the highest grade of oils. These oils are unique:

   - They are pure. Nothing is added to them. They are the result of simply distilling the plant.

   - They change with the environment. There is natural adjustment built into them based on the weather patterns and climate conditions of that season. Whereas the flu strain is always reacting to a flu shot (which is created in a lab by scientists based on what they think the flu will be like that season), oils have a built-in deterrence. Whereas the flu can morph to match a vaccination; it can't morph to match nature. Nature is always in transition.

   - Therapeutic grade oils do what other oils (lesser oils) won't do, because...

      - They are created with more care, with the intention of preserving the life of the plant.

      - They are the actual life source of the plant. When you use them, you are using something that is actually alive.

- Many people who have tried essential oils for *therapeuo* and reported that "they don't work" are actually reporting that aromatherapy grade and recreational grade oils don't work. If you try a lesser oil you will *not* get the benefits you will receive from a therapeutic grade oil.[78]

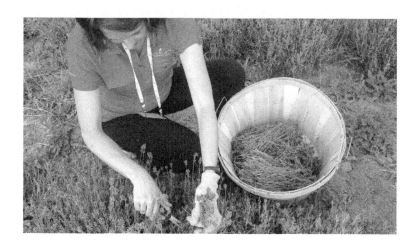

4. __Quality__ matters, particularly when we understand what a __Biblical__ __anointing__ actually is.

- **Consider the touching and the oils involved in a Biblical anointing.**

  - The touch was more than a simple, light touch.

---

[78] The production process includes far more than just the production of the oil. It includes the entire planting and harvesting process. Plants grown with pesticides, herbicides, and chemicals aren't pure- each of these actually migrate into the plant, altering its makeup. As well, some manufacturers will distill oils at a higher temperature (so that the process is faster and, therefore, cheaper). Others will undergo excessive distillations of the plant, using the raw material over and over- even after the life of the plant has already been used. In other words, its possible to have a great plant, but then compromise the life of it. So, therapeutic grade oils take the entire process- from the seed going into the ground all the way to the seal going onto the bottle- into consideration.

- To *anoint* means "to rub" or "to smear."[79]

- "... the Biblical references in Mark and James where healing take place with prayer, laying on of hands, and anointment with oils... the Biblical meaning of the word 'anoint' means 'to massage or rub with oil.'"[80]

- In other words, the touch wasn't a simple touch any more than baptism means to "flick a little bit of water on someone" (*baptizo* means "to submerge").

- This is an intimate sort of touching- thoroughly appropriate but *connecting*.

ANOINT

"TO RUB" -OR- "TO SMEAR"

- An anointing of any type most often included a large amount of oil.

  - Remember the "excessive" amount of oil that flowed down the beard of the priests, per Psalm 133:2?

  - Remember the amount of oil used on Jesus, when the woman anointed Him (see Matthew 26:7, Mark 14:3)?

---

[79] *Healing Oils of the Bible*, p6.

[80] *Healing Oils of the Bible*, p xxiii.

- Remember that Jesus actually rubbed mud over a blind man's eyes when anointing him and laying hands on him (John 9:6)? It was enough dirt and substance to actually make mud...

- An anointing might happen on the head, on the shoulders, on the hands, or even the feet (as in the instance of Jesus).[81]

> AN ANOINTING OF ANY TYPE MOST OFTEN INCLUDED A LARGE AMOUNT OF OIL.

- The touch- and the oil- would be noticeable to any bystanders.[82]

- **The smell would be predominant... so consider the role the limbic system plays in the process here.**

  - When you breathe, oil molecules move to the back passages of your nose, to the amygdala- the central headquarters of the limbic system. "The limbic system manages your storage for all of your emotional experiences."[83] This is why you can smell something- Fall leaves, apple pie, etc.- and a memory instantly arises in your soul. And, it's why hearing a certain song will instantly transport you back to a different time and place...

---

[81] For those familiar with the technique, the "raindrop" could actually be called an anointing if married to Scripture and/or prayer.

[82] Various verses throughout the Bible show that the Holy Spirit covers people when He anoints them. In some way, the oil would be similar. See Psalm 2:2, Lamentations 4:20, Ezekiel 28:14, Habakkuk 3:13, Zechariah 4:14, Luke 4:18, Acts 4:27, Acts 10:38, 2 Corinthians 1:21, 1 John 2:27.

[83] *Healing Oils of the Bible*, p24.

- Notably, the limbic system responds to words, smells, sound... all sensory input- yet, it doesn't have the capacity to communicate with language.[84]

- **The limbic system may also hold the key to understanding why you- or someone you know- has body aches and pains without any explanation or definable diagnosis!**

  - "When you have an emotional experience, especially a traumatic or painful one, the amygdala assigns a part of your body to remember the experience until you are ready to deal with it."[85]

  > THE LIMBIC SYSTEM MAY ALSO HOLD THE KEY TO UNDERSTANDING WHY YOU- OR SOMEONE YOU KNOW- HAS BODY ACHES AND PAINS WITHOUT ANY EXPLANATION OR DEFINABLE DIAGNOSIS!

  - "Repressed emotions are unfinished business" in the body, in other words. They can- and will- cause health malfunctions.[86]

  - The systemic malfunction might show up in the heart, the intestines... or a specific joint or muscle or organ. If you have an ache- for no known reason- you could be suppressing something.[87]

---

[84] A few more points about the limbic system: Dreams originate in the limbic system. Spiritual understanding occurs in the limbic system- not the assessment of facts and information, but revelation and intimacy. This is why it's difficult to sometimes communicate an encounter you've had with the Lord- and why it "falls flat" when you try to explain it to others. Words can't do it justice, because the limbic brain has such a greater capacity than words (re: revelation), while simultaneously having no capacity for written or spoken language.

[85] *Healing Oils of the Bible*, p25.

[86] *Healing Oils of the Bible*, p116.

[87] *Healing Oils of the Bible*, p116.

The Limbic Brain is One of the Deepest Parts

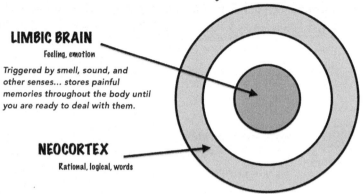

LIMBIC BRAIN
Feeling, emotion

Triggered by smell, sound, and other senses... stores painful memories throughout the body until you are ready to deal with them.

NEOCORTEX
Rational, logical, words

Notes: The Limbic Brain, which deals with emotions and smells, is the deepest part of the brain and manages memories for your body. When you use pure, therapeutic grade essential oils, you are touching this area, which is why they can act- and heal- on the emotional and spiritual level.

- **The limbic brain, which is the seat of emotions and feelings, is the "deepest" part of your brain.**

  - The limbic brain has no capacity for expressing itself in words, which is why it's often difficult to communicate your deepest feelings. Or, why you may feel like you're not explaining yourself well when you try to discuss your deepest feelings with someone.[88] Or, why outlining your dream in your mind or

---

[88] Simon Sinek, *Start With Why*, p56. He says this is why we have a difficult time explaining why we love our spouses- or why it's hard to relay a truly touching experience to someone else that wasn't there. The part of our brain that hardwired the memory (or the relationship) simply doesn't have the capacity to communicate those feelings. He writes, "When a decision feels right, we have a hard time explaining why we did what we did..." And, "It's not an accident that we use feel to explain those decisions, either" (p57). This graphic is adapted from Sinek, as well.

on paper actually supercharges you- yet you feel it "falls flat" when you try to describe it to a group of friends.

- The neocortex (frontal lobe of the brain), on the other hand, provides logic and reasoning... and is rich in words.

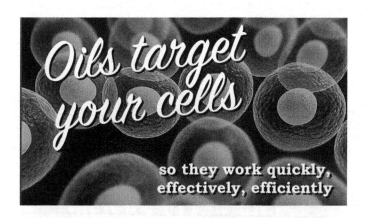

5. __How__ & __why__ essential oils work (four more reasons that quality matters).

- **First, essential oils are concentrated and small.** They are tiny, yet are power-packed!

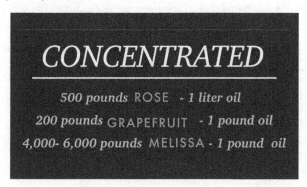

- It takes *a lot* of plant material to get a little oil.

    - 500 pounds of rose = 1 kilo of oil (about a liter)

    - 200 pounds of grapefruit 1.5 pounds of oil

    - 2-3 tons of Melissa = 1 pound of oil

- That's a lot of raw material (particularly when you remember that you're not cutting the oil with synthetics- but *only* using the plants), but you have the life / essence of all of those plants in that small amount of oil.

- The result is that "essential oils are 100 to 10,000 times more concentrated than herbs."[89]

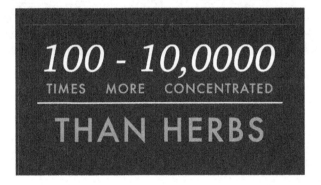

- The oil molecules are small enough to slide in and out of cells: "Essential oils have the unique ability to penetrate cell membranes and diffuse throughout the blood and tissues."[90]

- On the other hand, synthetics (recreational grade and aromatherapy grade oils) are larger, heavier, and cannot

---

[89] *Core Vigor and Vitality*, p3.

[90] *Essential Oil Pocket Reference*, page unknown.

travel. (Nor or they as potent, since they have a lot of "fillers" in them.)

- "To administrate healing at a cellular level the molecules of an oil must be tiny enough to penetrate into minute spaces. All of the molecules of essential oils are small enough to penetrate human skin, enter the blood stream through the alveolar cells of the lungs, and pass through the blood-brain barrier as well. All of the molecules of essential oils are also tiny enough to act as chemical messengers, unlocking the receptor sites of cells, and communicating with cellular intelligence as the level of the DNA. Molecules of such sizes, all less than 500 amu, are also aromatic and volatile."[91]

- **Second, the essential oil molecules out-number the cells in your body- *dramatically.***

  - Dr. David Stewart suggests each drop of oil contains 40 million trillion molecules.[92] That's a 4 with 19 zeros after it. It looks like:

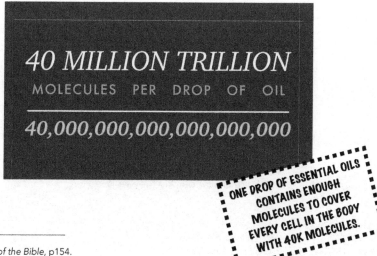

40 MILLION TRILLION
MOLECULES PER DROP OF OIL

40,000,000,000,000,000,000

ONE DROP OF ESSENTIAL OILS CONTAINS ENOUGH MOLECULES TO COVER EVERY CELL IN THE BODY WITH 40K MOLECULES.

---

[91] *Healing Oils of the Bible*, p154.

[92] *Healing Oils of the Bible*, pp27-28

- Compare the composition of our bodies: "we have 100 trillion cells… a lot." When you look at how many molecules are in each drop- that's right, a single drop- of essential oil, you get a better perspective. Stewart continues that "one drop of oil contains enough molecules to cover every cell in our body with 40,000 molecules."[93]

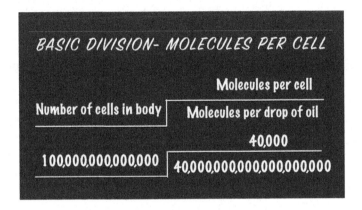

- When you remember that it only takes *one drop* in the right place at the right time for the right cell to communicate with the rest of your body, you can see just how profound the effects of a pure oil can be.

- **Third, essential oils travel.** "When applied to the body by rubbing on the feet, essential oils travel throughout the body and affect every cell, including the hair, within 20 minutes."[94]

  - Here is how quickly they work:

---

[93] David Stewart, *Healing Oils of the Bible*, pp27-28.

[94] See *Aromatherapy*, Gary Young, p21.

- *20-30 seconds,* the oils have move from the skin and enter the blood stream

- *20-30 minutes,* they have circulated throughout the entire body

- *2-3 hours,* they have been metabolized by the body

- Our bodies assimilate essential oils easily because when they are applied to the skin, inhaled, or even taken internally, they target our bodies' cells to act quickly, efficiently, and effectively.[95]

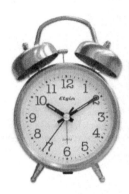

Essential Oils Act Fast!

20-30 SECONDS	The oils have moved from the skin and entered the blood stream
20-30 MINUTES	They have circulated throughout the entire body
2-3 HOURS	They have been metabolized by the body

- **Fourth, the oils communicate on the cellular level as they travel.** As they do, they clear up bad receptor sites, deprogram bad cells, and reprogram them. They can actually open receptor sites, push out the bad data, and rewrite code to heal DNA.

  - *Clear up bad receptor sites.* This allows information to pass. Your cells are constantly communicating with each other- and the rest of your body. This works in much the same way that antennas and cell phone towers work. If they're down,

---

95 In the next point we'll discuss three ways to use essential oils.

information doesn't pass.[96] Radios go silent; phone calls get dropped.

- *Deprogram bad info.* Not only does the message get through (because the receptor sites are clear), but the bad information in the cells gets eliminated. This is powerful- especially when you consider that cancer occurs when cells multiply with bad information.[97]

- *Reprogram good info.* For optimal health, your cells must continue multiplying. It's important that they do so in the right way, however. Replicating a damaged cell creates an exponentially increasing problem! Essential oils actively reprogram them with good information.[98]

4 Characteristics of Essential Oils

OILS ARE....	THIS MEANS THAT...
1. CONCENTRATED & SMALL	It takes a lot of raw material to make a pure oil, but once you have that drop of oil you have the life of all of those plants.
2. OUT-NUMBER THE CELLS IN YOUR BODY	It doesn't take much to do it's work. Just a few drops can accomplish the work required to touch the entire body.
3. TRAVEL THROUGHOUT THE BODY	They can be applied anywhere and will move everywhere, doing what needs to be done.
4. COMMUNICATE ON THE CELLULAR LEVEL	They are active and alive. They aren't just symbolic; they begin doing their work and actually achieve something.

[96] Study "phenols" for more information on this characteristic of essential oils.

[97] Study "sesquiterpenes" for more on this topic.

[98] Study "monoterpenes" for more on this topic.

- In other words, **when anointing someone with oil, we are doing far more than just "touching" them physically.** We are:

  - *Expressing to them that they are important and loved- through touch.* And, now we understand that far more is communicated through touch than we might have imagined possible.[99]

    > OILS COMMUNICATE ON THE CELLULAR LEVEL AS THEY TRAVEL... AND CLEAR UP BAD RECEPTOR SITES, DEPROGRAM BAD INFO, AND REPROGRAM GOOD INFO.

  - *We are offering them something helpful for the body.*

  - *And, this is before we have even prayed! In the next step we will invite God's supernatural power to do it's work!*

  - In other words, this isn't a symbolic- any more than baptism, communion, and laying on of hands is symbolic. There is more happening than we see- and we expect physical results to manifest!

NOT SYMBOLIC *ACTUAL*

- * BAPTISM
- * COMMUNION
- * LAYING ON HANDS
- * ANOINT TO HEAL

---

[99] Review "the healing power of touch" earlier in the book.

HOW &WHY

* CONCENTRATED & SMALL

* OUT-NUMBER YOUR CELLS

* TRAVEL

* COMMUNICATE WITH CELLS

AS THEY TRAVEL

* CLEAN BAD RECEPTOR SITES

* CLEAR UP BAD INFO

* REPLACE WITH GOOD INFO

6. There are three ways you can use essential oils-
__touching__, __breathing__, or __swallowing__.

- **First, you may rub them on your skin and let them do their thing.** Your skin is the largest organ in your body. So, it's hard to "miss" with this one.

  - For instance, Cristy J. writes, "We just used lavender the other day when our toddler ran head into the corner of the wall. He was so upset and crying. Momma whipped out our lavender straight away and applied it to his boo-boo. It calmed him and soothed his sweet wittle skin."

  - "Anointing" in the Bible is an example of *touching*.

- **Second, you may breathe them.** Your skin is your largest organ, but your sense of smell is the strongest sense we have. It's tied to the limbic system, where memories and feelings are stored. This is why essential oils can support your mood and heal emotional wounds!

- Shannon M. says, "I love to use Frankincense... before starting my work weekend. It helps ground me & get me ready for a busy day."

- In the Bible we see Aaron offer incense after Korah's rebellion (see Numbers 16). We also see holy incense in the Temple (we'll discuss it in more detail later in the book).[100]

- **Third, you may swallow them.** That is, you may actually take them orally- by using a capsule, by dropping the oils in your drink, or by simply placing a few drops under your tongue.

  - Rachel R. recalls her daughter's grumpy tummy: "The school was calling me to get her every day. She was so unhapppy. She took capsules of DiGize and Peppermint diluted with coconut oil. After trying for months to get her better with traditional methods- to no avail- in just a few short weeks with Young Living her tummy was supported back to its natural healthy digestion!"

  - Jesus was offered wine mingled with Myrrh on the Cross (Matthew 27:33)

Three Ways You Can Use Essential Oils

YOU CAN...	THIS MEANS THAT YOU...
TOUCH THEM	Apply them directly to your skin
BREATHE THEM	Smell them
SWALLOW THEM	Put them in a capsule, place a few drops in your mouth, or put a few drops in your favorite drink (tea or water)

[100] This is a powerful idea. Smell literally "takes you back" in time to a memory. This means that anytime you smelled the plants that were present in the Holy Incense, it would instantly remind you of your Father's presence. You would literally sense fingerprints of His proximity throughout the world.

7. We see all three methods **throughout** the __Bible__.

- *Touch-* apply essential oils directly to your skin.

- *Breathe-* inhale essential oils by using smelling them straight from the bottle, cupping them in your hand, or using a diffuser.

- *Swallow / ingest-* place a few drops in your mouth, put the oils in a capsule, or add a few drops to water or tea.

Selected Examples of all 3 Methods in Scripture

HOW	EXAMPLE(S)
TOUCH THEM	The Good Samaritan (Luke 10:34)
	Isaiah 1:6 speaks of oils being applied to wounds, bruises, and scars
	Esther treated her skin with myrrh for 6 months, leading to her night with the king (Esther 2:12)
	Leviticus 14:17 outlines protocol for treating leprosy. Notably, the right hand and thumb (which are referenced are the pituitary point on the Vitaflex chart)
BREATHE THEM	The Holy Incense inside the Tabernacle (Exodus 30:8, 34:6)
	Korah's rebellion (Number 16:46-50)
	At Passover, the crushing leaves of the hyssop branch would release the hyssop fragrance (see Exodus 12:22)
SWALLOW THEM	Wine with myrrh was offered to Jesus on the Cross.

C. Essential oils move you __higher__, __faster__.

1. Different kinds of __frequency__ exist- __frequency__ being "the measurable rate of __electrical__ __energy__ flow that is constant between two points").

- A.C. / *alternating current*- most appliances in the home use alternating current ("things made by man").[101]

- D.C. / *direct current*- plants, animals, and people all have a frequency ("things made by God").

Two Kinds of Frequency

	AKA	DISTINCTION
A.C.	Alternating Current	Things made by man (appliances)
D.C.	Direct Current	Things made by God (plants, animals, people)

2. Your __frequency__ drops as your state of __health__ drops. Frequency, then, is a measure of how __alive__ you- or anything else- is.

---

[101] For more on frequency see Gary Young's *Aromatherapy*, p81.

- **Notice the progression- a lower frequency means you aren't doing as well; a higher frequency means you're more alive.**[102] Again, everything has a frequency. *Everything.* Everything, well, except dead things, that is.[103] Frequency is defined as "the measurable rate of electrical energy flow that is constant between any two points."[104]

    - A healthy human has a standing frequency of 62-68 MHz. As your state of health drops, so does that frequency. Your frequency is a measure of how strong and "alive" you really are.[105]

    - Cold symptoms manifest around 58 MHz, as at this point your immune system begins shutting down.[106]

    - Flu symptoms surface around 57 MHz.

    - Candida appears around 55 MHz.

    - Cancer *can* begin when the body falls below 42 MHz.

    - The process of dying begins about 25 MHz and bottoms at at 0 MHz when you are pronounced dead.

> A LOWER FREQUENCY MEANS YOU AREN'T DOING AS WELL; A HIGHER FREQUENCY MEANS YOU'RE MORE ALIVE.

---

[102] See Gary Young's *Aromatherapy*, p38f., for this discussion. Also, see *Healing Oils of the Bible*, p32f.

[103] This is not a new idea. In fact, you're familiar with it. "In 1924, William Einthoven received a Nobel Prize for his discovery that heart electricity could rerecorded with a galvanometer. In the 1970s, magnetometers were developed that could measure brain fields. Now, the electrocardiogram (ECG) and electroencephalogram (EEG) are standard tools for medical diagnosis." See p160-161 in *The Physics of Heaven*, by Judy Franklin and Ellyn Davis.

[104] Gary Young, *Aromatherapy*, p35. See also *The Physics of Heaven*. Discoveries in Quantum Physics suggest that "everything that exists is, in its essence, energy" (p112).

[105] This list comes from *Healing Oils of the Bible*, p32. See also Gary Young, *Aromatherapy*, p38.

[106] Gary Young, *Aromatherapy*, p38.

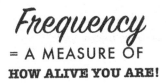

62-68 MHz = Healthy

58 MHz = Cold symptoms manifest

57 MHz = Flu symptoms

55 MHz = Candida

42 MHz = Cancer can begin

25 MHz = Process of dying begins

0 MHz = Death

- You probably understand this more than you think you do. **Some days, you feel more energetic and vibrant. Other days, you feel like your dragging... sluggish.** Your frequency- the measure of how "alive" you are- is higher / lower on different days.

- **Research shows the following boosting your frequency to a higher level has amazing health benefits.**

  - Royal Raymond Rife, a medical doctor who studied human frequencies in the early 1900s, discovered that he could actually *destroy* viruses and cancer cells at certain frequencies. He found that other frequencies prevented the development of disease.[107]

  - *What does this have to do with essential oils?* Well, here's the kicker: "Clinical research shows that essential oils have the highest frequency of any natural substance known to man, creating an environment in which disease, bacteria, virus, fungus, etc., *cannot* live."[108] Notice, those things *cannot* live.

---

[107] Gary Young, *Aromatherapy*, p35.

[108] Gary Young, *Aromatherapy*, p40.

Not, "they prefer something else… so they can't thrive" but they *cannot even exist.*

- **Notice the frequencies of selected essential oils in the chart below, and how they help maintain a higher frequency.[109]**

Frequencies of Selected Oils

ESSENTIAL OIL	FREQUENCY / MHZ
Rose	320 MHz
Helichrysum	181 MHz
Lavender	118 MHz
Blue Tansy	105 MHz
German Chamomile	105 MHz
Juniper	98 MHz
Peppermint	78 MHz
Basil	52 MHz

- The numbers are astounding.[110] You'll see that the frequency of rose is about *five times* the frequency of a healthy human. Peppermint, a very commonly used oil (it's relatively inexpensive and easy to get) is a full 10 MHz *higher* than a healthy reading of 62-68 MHz. No wonder it gets people jazzed up![111]

- The frequency of the oils is one of the reasons that the pain "goes away" almost immediately in many cases within a few minutes of applying certain oils. Quite simply, a lower

[109] Of course, now we're coming back to the quality issue!

[110] This information comes from *Healing Oils of the Bible*, p33.

[111] Do you have any Peppermint nearby? Open it up…

personal frequency means you are not feeling well- and all the symptoms of not feeling well (like pain) come with that.

- "One of the most important healing modalities of the oils is their ability to lift our bodily frequencies to levels where disease cannot exist."[112] Since an essential oil can raise your frequency, though, you start feeling better as your frequency elevates.

- "Essential oils have vibrational frequencies that match and are believed to enhance the vibrational frequency of healthy cells in your body."[113]

- This, of course, goes back to the "quality issue" we discussed earlier. "Dead oils cannot heal. They may still have a fragrance or flavor to satisfy the perfumers or food makers, but they are not therapeutic grade oils."[114]

Higher Frequency
= YOU'RE STRONGER
+ ILLNESS / DISEASE
CANNOT EXIST

Lower Frequency
= YOU'RE WEAKER
+ ILLNESS / DISEASE
THRIVE!

---

[112] *Healing Oils of the Bible*, p33.

[113] See "Good Vibrations," Chapter 6 in *The Physics of Heaven*. Go to p62.

[114] *Healing Oils of the Bible*, p180.

- **As you might expect, healthier foods have higher frequencies.**

  - On a side note, foods have frequencies, too. David Stewart writes, "fresh herbs measure 20-27 MHz... fresh produce 5-10 MHz. Processed or canned food measured zero. In other words, there is no life or life force in canned or processed foods."

  - Now you have a scientific answer (another one) when your kids ask you why you don't like McDonald's. And you know why you feel like junk when you eat too much pizza. After learning about frequencies it's not hard to believe the old but true adage, "You are what you eat."

  - Yes, a lifestyle of *therapeuo* includes the foods you eat.[115]

  - Remember what Hippocrates said: "Let food be your medicine and medicine be your food."

Frequency = A MEASURE OF **HOW ALIVE YOUR** *food is!*

20 - 27 MHz = Some plants and herbs

5 - 10 MHz = Other plants and herbs

0 MHz = Processed & canned

[115] Yes, Paul did say, "Eat what is set before you without asking questions" (1 Corinthians 10:25.; see also 8:4f.). But, he was talking about meat sacrificed to idols- not junk food. Junk food is toxic. And, it happens loads of empty calories. This means there is no nutritional value to give your body the energy it needs. In other words, it adds toxins while creating deficiencies- at the same time. Because you are consuming calories, you will gain weight. Because the calories are synthetic and not natural, your body is unable to digest them- so they convert largely to fat. All calories are not created equal. You can be obese- and literally starving- at the same time. A lot of people are. I was one of them!

- **Now, at this point, you might wonder:** *Why not just pray?*

    - In a moment we will discuss prayer- and how it drives health and wholeness. Remember, though, we are looking for a lifestyle of *therapeuo* (even as we pray for *iaomai* to occur).

        > PRAYER AND OILS- AND OTHER FORMS OF THERAPEUO- ACTUALLY WORK TOGETHER AND ENHANCE EACH OTHER.

    - We will see that prayer and oils- and other forms of *therapeuo*- actually work together and enhance each other. "Each increases the power of the other such that their combined ability to heal is greater than the sum of the two... When we pray over the oils, their frequencies increase."[116]

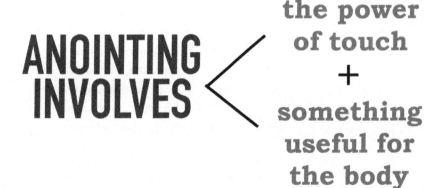

ANOINTING INVOLVES < the power of touch + something useful for the body

---

[116] *Healing Oils of the Bible*, p93.

3. This does not mean that we abandon _ **modern medicine** _; we do, however, need to evaluate it honestly.

- **First, the issue of modern medicine raises an interesting question about where we place our faith.** "Christians [often] exhibit more faith in secular medicine than in God and prayer, yet they object to God's medicine (oils), saying that prayer is sufficient and they don't need oils."[117]

- **Second, we can make a better decision when we understand what medicine actually does to our body.** Particularly, let's evaluate what pharmaceuticals do as well as what antibiotics do.[118] The short version is this:

    - *Pharmaceuticals target symptoms and create chaos!*

        - Symptoms are not illnesses, however. Rather, symptoms are there to tell you something is wrong. Symptoms are messengers. Remember, the limbic brain may store a harmful memory somewhere in your body, which may manifest as a symptom. You don't unplug the "check engine" bulb on your dash board- you take the car to the shop to have it repaired. Pharmaceuticals never address the real issue. In effect, they kill the messenger (the symptom) that is alerting you that something is wrong.

        - This can be a great thing- and was designed to be a *temporary* relief while deeper issues were handled. For instance, our youngest daughter Miriam

---

[117] *Healing Oils of the Bible*, p93.

[118] Learn more about pharmaceuticals on p46f. and more about antibiotics on p74f. of *Healing Oils of the Bible*.

fractured her wrist. She was given Motrin to deal with the pain while the doctor took care of her broken bone. We did *not* give her Motrin to cover the pain... to simply cover the pain... and continue covering the pain. We covered the pain only so that we could address the deeper issue.[119]

- As a result, these drugs simply lie to your body.[120] Because of this, the symptom simply moves elsewhere, manifesting as a different ache or pain. This is why people often find themselves continually adjusting their meds once they get on them. Why? Because the messenger is fighting to get your attention![121]

- Medicines also introduce toxins into your body. And, remember, at the base level, the root cause of all dis-ease is either a *toxin* (the presence of something that shouldn't be in your body) or a *deficiency* (the absence of something that should be). They are a

---

[119] So you could originally deal with a surface symptom, then drive down deep at the underlying issue. You might medicate high blood pressure *temporarily*, so that you could deal with the entire cardiovascular system- or discern what else might be happening. The problem is two-fold, now: *First, permanence.* We don't medicate temporarily. We medicate permanently. Drug companies don't make money if you get well and cease taking their drugs. *Second, the weakest link.* Your body is a system. Whenever one point of exit (for the messenger) is blocked, it moves to the next weakest point of exposure. Think of this like a faulty chain. The weakest link snaps first. We repair it and then add more weight to the load. So the next weakest link snaps. We repair and add more weight... so another link snaps... The goal is not to continue repairing chain links, however. The goal is to remove the weight which causes the links to snap!

[120] Note what John 8:44 says about the "lying" issue.

[121] Here's an example: If I really, really need to get in touch with my Dad, I'll call his cell phone. If that doesn't work, I'll call his home phone. If I can't get him there, I'll reach out to my mom... then my sister... This is how symptoms work in your body. If you kill one (i.e., smash the cell phone), another one pops up (the home phone). Your body is trying desperately to communicate with you!

medical intervention that changes the outcome of anything that was happening…[122]

- Many of the issues we see today are a result of toxins. For instance, many people take Zoloft or Prozac for depression (which is caused by low levels of serotonin- a natural chemical your body releases when you feel loved and accepted). Impotence is a side effect of both drugs. Enter Viagra.[123] Of course, this might cause sleepless nights, so enter Ambien- a drug for sleep. This makes the medicated person tired and sexually disinterested… which gives rise to further feelings of depression… creating a huge cycle.

- *Antibiotics target bacteria- but kill everything good and bad!*

  - Because they target good and bad bacteria, not making a distinction between the two (your gut has healthy flora, good bacteria which aid in digestion, for instance), they begin wiping out your entire system.[124]

  - They offer no help for viruses (flu, cold). And, they also have a limited duration of functional time. The bad bacteria get smarter and actually "immunize" themselves to the antibiotic.

---

[122] Another example: childbirth. Sometimes, interventions (i.e., C-section, induction, etc.) are necessary. Many times- most of the time- they are not. When we introduce them, though, we change outcomes. Induction with drugs causes contractions to be more intense that natural contractions. And they may come too soon. They may result in a C-section- when the mother wanted a vaginal delivery. Does this mean sections are bad? No. Sometimes, they are necessary. But, we change outcomes when we add factors to the mix.

[123] This was produced by the company to originally market to their clients who were already on anti-depressants!

[124] Chemotherapy does the same thing. It kills every cell in the body- like a "wipe" on the hard drive of your computer.

- If masking symptoms with a pharmaceutical drug is akin to removing the check engine light in your car instead of investigating the problem, antibiotics are the equivalent of smashing the entire engine- when it may simply be an oil filter or spark plug that needs to be addressed.[125]

How Modern Medicine Works

	GOES FOR...	SO THEY...
Pharmaceuticals (Prescription drugs are, strangely enough, the 3rd leading cause of death in the U.S.- behind heart disease and cancer)	**Symptoms** They never address the real issue. In effect, they kill the messenger (the symptom) that is alerting you that something is wrong.	Lie to your body. Because of this, the symptom simply moves elsewhere, manifesting as a different ache or pain. This is why people often find themselves continually adjusting their meds once they get on them. (Note what John 8:44 says about the "lying" issue).
Antibiotics	**Bacteria only** Because they target good and bad bacteria, not making a distinction between the two (your gut has healthy flora, good bacteria which aid in digestion, for instance), they begin wiping out your system.	They offer no help for viruses (flu, cold). They kill everything- good and bad. They have a limited duration of functional time. The bad bacteria get smarter and actually "immunize" themselves to the antibiotic.

[125] Unless you address the body system that needs support, you're not making long-term progress. I know of people- I'm sure you do, too- who went to the hospital and only got sicker. I know of a few who even did so and died! Again, you're dealing with a symptom- not the actual issue.

- Third, understanding the Biblical background of the word and concept of *pharmaceutical* sheds some light on how these drugs work- and what they do.

  - The root word is revealing:

    - Pharmaceutical = *Pharmakeuein* in Greek (the language of the New Testament)

    - Poison = *Pharmakon*

    - *Pharmakon* is also translated as "witchcraft" and "sorcery."

"NOW THE WORKS OF THE FLESH ARE EVIDENT, WHICH ARE: ENVY, HATRED, STRIFE, LUST, DISSENSIONS, PHARMAKON..."

– Galatians 5:19-21

PHARMACEUTICAL

Pharmakon (Greek)

TRANSLATED AS

POISON · WITCHCRAFT · SORCERY

- In addition, several Bible verses provide insight:

  - In Revelation 9:21, 18:23, 21:8, and 22:15 John refers to sorcery- and uses derivatives of the words above in each instance.

  - When Paul recounts the "works of the flesh" he writes: "Now the works of the flesh are evident: sexual immorality, impurity, sensuality, idolatry, sorcery, enmity, strife, jealousy, fits of anger, rivalries, dissensions, divisions, envy, drunkenness, orgies, and things like these..." (Galatians 5:19-21 ESV). In this passage, sorcery is also *pharmakon*.

- In other words, pharmaceuticals are a work of the flesh- *they are man's attempts to bring healing*.[126] Remember, though, healing is something that has already been given by the blood of Jesus (*iaomai*), and it is our pattern for living now (*therapeuo*). Plus, His healing encompasses every area of life (*sozo*).

- Perhaps this explains where there are over 106,000 deaths per year as a direct result of FDA approved drugs! (Prescription drugs are, strangely enough, the 3rd leading

---

[126] Yes, the flesh is present when we sin in the typical sense of defiance or disobedience. However, the flesh also appears when we seek to do a good thing in our own strength by striving for it, instead of accomplishing the task in God's power. When we do something ourselves rather than allowing the Spirit of God to manifest it for us, we've walked in the flesh.

Now, this doesn't mean we don't participate in what God is doing. *Therapeuo* requires our participation. Think about the walls of Jericho (Joshua 6). God clearly won the battle. He brought down the walls- when the people shouted after walking around the city a few times. They participated, but it was clearly His battle and His victory.

Our "flesh" ways of handling health have ventured us into an area of "disease management" rather than wholeness and healing. Why? There's not much money in Divine healing or *therapeuo*!

cause of death in the U.S.- behind heart disease and cancer.)[127]

- **Fourth, there is a place for modern medicine. But we need to understand what it is...**

  - If oils work- *without* the side effects- the question arises as to why drug companies *won't* manufacture them. Here's why: drug companies seek "pharmacological purity."

    - This means every drug they make will be exactly like every other drug of the same kind. They can test them and get the same results over and over.

    - Because oils occur in nature (they come from plants) and because nature cannot be controlled (the plants will change depending on the climate, that season's precipitation, the time of harvest, etc.), the oils will *never* have "pharmacological purity."[128] You can't patent mother nature.

    - Drug companies are seeking *customers*- not cures or success stories.

  - I am not suggesting that you don't go to the doctor or that you neglect using medicines. However, I think we can agree that sorcery, witchcraft, and poison are *not* what Jesus

---

[127] In the US, we have 5% of the world's population, but consume 75% of the world's prescription drugs. More people die of these drugs- all sold legally- each year than die of car accidents. 10% of Americans are on antidepressants. Oddly enough. the death rate for illegal street drugs doesn't even make the top 10, according to *USA Today* and *Time*. Source: *Prescription Thugs*, a 2015 documentary film by Chris Bell.

Ironically, many legal drugs are actually repacked creations of street drugs. Ritalin and Aderhol are remarkably similar to Meth. Opiates (and Oxys) are derivatives of Heroine. It was shocking how many people I met during my days running a rehabilitation center that stumbled into addiction via prescription drugs that were remarkable approximations of their "street" counterparts.

[128] Actually, recreational grade and aromatherapy grade essential oils will have pharmacological purity. They are created in a lab with synthetics. On the other hand, therapeutic grade oils never will have it. It's impossible to tame what our Father continues creating on our behalf! We discussed this earlier in the book.

intended when He said, "I've come that you might have life more abundantly..." (John 10:10).

- "When a genuine medical emergency exists and the threat of death is near, a shot of antibiotics or the application of an allopathic procedure may save your life..."[129]

- Just this past year we visited the doctor for broken bones (including a surgery and an overnight stay), well visits (read: checkups) and even orthodontic work (though, I know, this is a different kind of doctor). We are not opposed to medical interventions. However, they are seen as temporary, short-term blessings- and are used to supplement our path of *therapeuo*. They are *not* used as ongoing crutches or as replacements for wise choices.

MODERN MEDICINE

- * **WHERE WE PLACE FAITH**
- * **HOW MODERN MEDICINE WORKS**
- * **BIBLICAL BACKGROUND**
- * **THE PLACE OF MODERN MEDICINE**

---

[129] *Healing Oils of the Bible*, p75.

4. Focus on living __*above*__ ___*the*___ ___*line*___ - at a higher frequency!

- **The Bible tells us where to focus:** "Whatever things are true, whatever things are noble, whatever things are just, whatever things are pure, whatever things are lovely, whatever things are of good report, if there is any virtue and if there is anything praiseworthy—meditate on these things" (Philippians 4:8).

- **This isn't just advice about our thoughts- this is for all of life, including health and wellness.**

  - A lifestyle of *therapeuo* focuses higher...

  - *Therapeuo* looks to *prevent* instead of fix, to *exercise* instead of remaining sedentary, and to address the body's *systems* rather than the body's symptoms.

Living above the wellness line

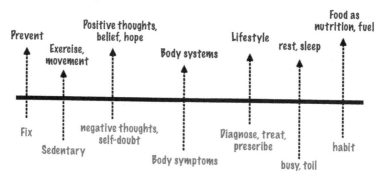

Notes: *We want to do things that push our bodies "above the line." Too often, people focus "below the line," looking at unwellness rather than looking at wellness. We are told to think on things that are pure, noble, true... (see Philippians 4:8).*

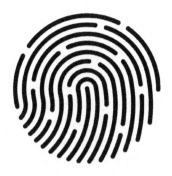

Apply Habit 2 & Touch

ESSENTIAL OILS IN THE BIBLE
ESSENTIAL OILS EXPLAINED
ESSENTIAL OILS MOVE YOU HIGHER, FASTER

☐ Symptoms are messengers from your body's systems trying to grab your attention- so that you can help your body, not simply deal with the symptom. When someone calls you on the telephone, you know that the person on the other end of the line is the most important part of the equation- not the phone itself, right? And, you know the adage "Don't shoot the messenger!"[130] What messages is your body sending you? Where have you paid more attention to the "phone" than the person (body) on the other end of the line? Where you have shot the messenger?

---

[130] Yes, I know the messenger usually tells us this when they are bringing us a message they know we won't like! Well, what about your body!?

☐ I wrote about forgiveness earlier in the book. I mentioned that many times people forgive and find they are instantly healed of an issue that's been bothering them. Here's why: the limbic system stores hurtful memories throughout your body until you are ready to deal with them. A hurtful memory may surface symptomatically as a physical ailment.[131] Remember, it's just a messenger, though. It's your body calling you, telling you to deal with something so that you can live well. So, let's do it... Who do you need to forgive for something?

Close your eyes, ask the Lord, and write their name and what you need to forgive them for doing. Then, release it to the Lord. (When we do this, we aren't saying that what they did wasn't wrong; we simply release the consequences to our Father, and set aside the weight we are carrying.)

☐ After doing the exercise above, what do you see, sense, or feel about your physical body?

---

[131] "The consequences of unforgiveness may bind you to a disease resulting from the sin of bitterness and unforgiveness" (see A More Excellent Way, p5).

APPLY HABIT 2 & TOUCH

☐ I mentioned, too, that many people were healed simply by uncovering their identity as a beloved child of a gracious and loving Heavenly Father. What is your spiritual identity? What is your Father like?

☐ Most health books I've read refer to the gut (digestion tract, etc.) as the "second brain." Many of these authors contend that by getting the stomach in good health (re: the food you eat) you can deal with most other health issues pretty quickly. This works in two predominant ways that I've seen personally. First, if we begin eating right, a lot of health issues that we've been tolerating simply disappear... *quickly*. Second, if you're carrying unforgiveness, anxiety and stress, or a delated spiritual identity, it may show up in your gut first... you may tend to over-eat to compensate... or you may develop and irritable bowel. What is your experience here? And what changes might you make...?

☐ Let's discuss pharmaceuticals and even over-the-counter meds. We tend to "cover" things up (messengers), so the body begins calling us from somewhere else. Another symptom pops up. I've got a theory about why pharmaceuticals have a long, long list of side effects- related to this. What if... *just what if...* the side effects they list are all of the messengers that popped up in clinical trials when the first messenger was covered? That is, what if the list of side effects is really various people's bodies calling them, alerting them to a deeper issue? Could it really be the limbic system switching to another "check engine light" in the soul?

☐ There's an amazing power in touch. It think it may be even more profound today- in our world of hyper-connectivity with the Internet, social media, and rampant texting. In many ways, we've gone for "shallow and wide" relationships instead of deep and meaningful ones. We're surrounded by people, yet many of us are alone. *What do you think about the power of touch?*

☐ What about the things that aren't explained in the Bible- things like baptism, communion, and anointing. *Are these symbolic acts only? Or does something powerful happen in the moment?* Does does this apply to essential oils? And why does the quality matter?

☐ How much money have you- or people in your family- spent on physicians? Are you being helped (because, yes, there is a place for medical professionals!), or are you like the woman whom Jesus healed, the one who'd spent all that she had on doctors but had not gotten better, had only gotten worse (see Mark 5:26)? This is the condition of many people today. What's your story?

☐ Why do you think people are hesitant to spend the money on better food? Exercise (i.e., a gym membership or a great pair of fitness shoes)? Why do we complain that we don't have time to take care of ourselves (i.e., exercise, prepare healthy foods), yet we have time for lengthy doctor visits (and even sick days) that might be eliminated with a lifestyle of *therapeuo*?

☐ Pastor Wright asks, "When we minister to someone and they are not healed, what do you think we ought to do? Make up a theology saying God does not heal today? Make up a theology that someone did not have enough faith? What do you think we ought to do?"[132] I'd love to know what you think we should do...

---

[132] *A More Excellent Way*, p39.

☐ Some people suggest God causes sickness and disease, that He inflicts His children with harm to refine them, teach them a lesson, or grow some other trait in them. What do you think? If God causes illness, wouldn't it make sense to not try and fight against it, but to just "tough it out" and learn the lesson? Or even to *enjoy* it? What are you learning in this book about God's character and the origin of sickness and disease?

☐ Share your thoughts on the following statement: "The oils are God's medicines."[133]

☐ Touch is used in several ways throughout Scripture. It seems to be so important that it's not just limited to healing. We see touch used to impart spiritual gifts to new leaders, to bless children, to impart the Holy Spirit...and to heal. In what ways might touch become a powerful force in your own life and / or ministry?

☐ We raised a few questions about the place of modern medicine in this chapter. I mentioned...

---

[133] Source unknown.

- We need to decide where we're really placing our faith...

- We need to be honest about what medicines do to our bodies...

- We need to understand the Biblical perspective of pharmaceuticals...

- We need to realize modern medicine can be an amazing blessing.

So, where is modern medicine's place in your life, in light of what we discussed?

☐ Review the three ways in which essential oils can be used. And make a few notes as to where you see them used in each way throughout the Bible.

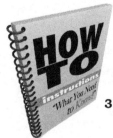

1. On your skin

2. Breathe them

3. Swallow them

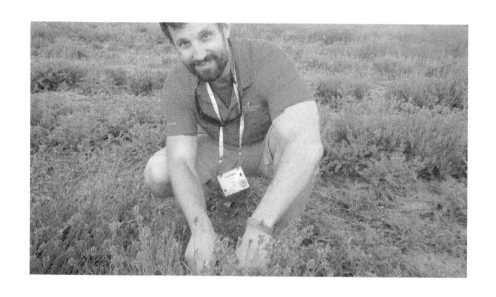

4. The Oils

WHAT DO YOU NEED?
THE OILS OF THE PREMIUM STARTER KIT
THE TWELVE OILS OF ANCIENT SCRIPTURE

"...He began to send them out two by two, and gave them power... So they went and preached... and they cast out many demons, and anointed with oil many who were sick, and healed them" (Mark 6:7,12,13 NKJV).

"You anoint my head with oil" (Psalm 23:5 NIV).

A. What do you __need__?

- As we mentioned earlier in the book, **many times God will do something *to* you before He does something *through* you. The greatest work you do for the Kingdom most often begins with the work He does in you!**

1. Think about ____your body____...

- **We've already addressed our beliefs.** So, let's move to the body...

- Before we move through the oils, I want to do a quick exercise. **Take a moment and think about your body and your health and make a list of the areas where you would like to see greater wellness and support.**

> MAKE A LIST OF THE AREAS WHERE YOU WOULD LIKE TO SEE GREATER WELLNESS AND SUPPORT.

- *Do you want to experience:*

  - *Improved digestion?*

  - *Immune system function?*

  - *Brain health?*

  - *Better sleep?*

  - *Improved mood?*

- Make a list of your top 3 priorities and keep it in mind while we are discussing the oils.

  - _____

  - _____

  - _____

2. What you'll __see__...

- **There are 11 oils in Young Living's Premium Starter Kit- 5 single oils and 6 blends.** We'll discuss the 5 single oils first, and then walk through the blends. The blends are combinations of single oils put together as a proprietary mixture because the synergy of some of the oils works so well together.

B. The oils of the __Premium__ __Starter__ __Kit__.

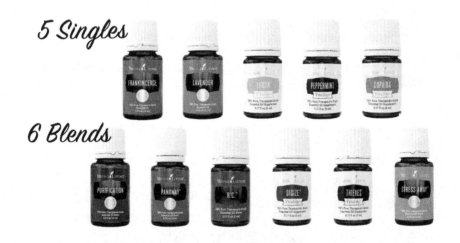

Above: the 11 most popular essential oils. This is a great place to begin, as it gives you a well-rounded set to address multiple facets of health and wellness- and even help around the home! White labels marked "Vitality" easily reference certain oils which may be ingested.

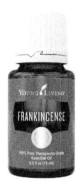

Frankincense is a soothing, uplifting, and valuable oil with a rich history- the wise men brought this one to baby Jesus! It's used to support the immune and respiratory systems, to brighten one's mood, and may even prove helpful for focus and brain function!

It's great to add to your skin care regimen- My wife loves how this one feels on her face!

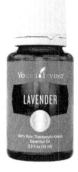

Let's talk about Lavender, which has a relaxing aroma that may improve sleep, reduce stress, calm the nerves, or even soothe fussy babies. Because it's so versatile, Lavender has a unique nick name.

Kelly F. says, "Lavender really is 'the Swiss Army knife of essential oils.' The kids even ask for it by that name, now."

What is it not good for?! We use it for relaxation, soothing skin, and even baking.

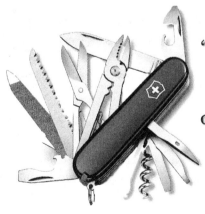

"Lavender really is the 'Swiss Army Knife' of essential oils. The kids even ask for it by that name, now!"

- Kelly F.

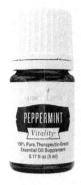

Peppermint facilitates heightened energy and awareness. This oil is an athlete's favorite. Many use it before a workout to enhance their oxygen levels!

Not an athlete? No problem- just use it for a natural "pick me up" whenever you need to stay- or get- alert! David O. says he uses Peppermint when driving late at night; others use it as an substitute for a bad coffee habit!

Peppermint is also prized for its ability to calm a grumpy stomach- it's really supportive to the digestive system.

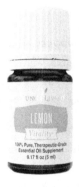

Lemon is a simple, versatile, powerful oil. It's pressed from the rind- not made from the juice. Lemon soothes the occasional sore throat, energizes the body when added to your favorite drink, and even acts as a natural "goo-remover" for those tough messes.

In the Bible we see oils used for houses, shields, furniture, and other physical items. Remember, everything is under God's domain and your stewardship- even your stuff!

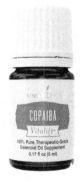

Copaiba was discovered by Gary Young, the founder of Young Living, in Ecuador. A soothing oil, this one is a mom's favorite, as it's helpful for teething babies when applied to their gums or outside of the jaw. And, it's uniquely one of the oils that enhances the effectiveness of other oils.

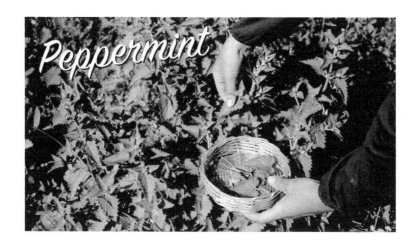

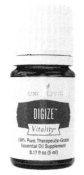

DiGize is the gold standard for digestive support. Whether you've eaten too much, if your dinner didn't quite agree with you, or if your stomach feels a bit rumbly, this is the "go to" for normal digestive support. We *never* leave home without it!

One mom writes, "When your toddler comes into your room with hand on tummy whining, 'I need die-die sh' you know the oils are making a difference! DiGize to the rescue!" And, yes, that Mom may be known for having a bottle in every room of her house!

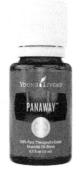

PanAway is another blend you don't want to be without, particularly for muscle and bone support.

Debbie C., a 63-year old grandmother of 13, says she keeps a bottle in her purse, one on her bedside table, another on her kitchen, and one in the van. She applies it to joints and muscles and gives it to her friends!

Of course, youngsters like it, too. Noah J., an 11-year old, uses it soothe normal growing pains, helping him sleep through the night comfortably.

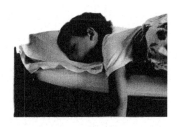

Purification is a popular blend to use in your home instead of chemically-laden air fresheners, scented candles, and aerosol sprays- all of which are being revealed to be harmful for you.

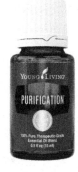

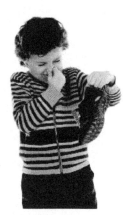

Kids with stinky feet and even stinkier shoes? Place a few drops of Purification on a cotton ball and toss the balls in the shoes. (Yeah, it's good to diffuse after these boys use the restroom, too.)

RC supports optimal respiratory function when applied to the chest. I went running with a few friends and found out my pal Verick liberally applied RC to his chest before the jog began. "I felt like he had cheated," I told the others, "he was running so strong!"

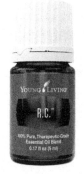

With singles like Eucalyptus and Peppermint in this blend, RC packs strong support for normal breathing at all times.

A high school teacher says, "I have been learning to use all sorts of combinations in my diffuser for my classroom. I took my diffuser home at one point and my high school students begged me to bring it back. They will even stand over it and try to breathe more of it in. They really love RC."

Ever leave the laundry in the washer a bit too long (long enough to get that nice, sour smell)? Re-run it with Purification added to the detergent... and presto!

Stress Away is... well... it's what it says!

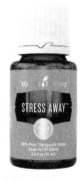

Ever had a stressful day? Long day at the office? Couldn't get the kids to totally fall in line? Maybe the person driving the car in front of you on the way here need to go back to driving school?

Place just a bit on your hands, cup them together, and take a deep breath. I promise you, this will be like taking a mini-vacation from your day...

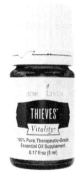

Thieves may actually be our favorite blend, though. Let me tell you where the name comes from. Apparently, during the Bubonic Plague that ravaged Europe, everyone was getting sick except for four thieves who were able to steal items from tombs and the dead & dying. Once caught, they were told they would be allowed to go free if they offered up the secret to their immunity. They revealed a concoction of essential oils- a blend upon which our Thieves oil is based. Unfortunately, the crooks were still executed, but society did take advantage of the new immunity recipe!

We aren't living in medieval Europe, but we come in contact with wellness detours at every turn. So, **we support ours and our kids growing bodies and developing immune systems with Thieves every single day.**

THE OILS

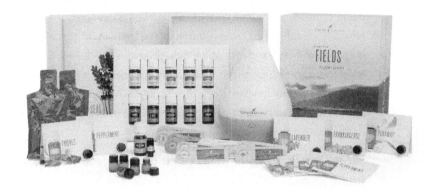

The Premium Starter Kit is the best way to get started. It includes 11 of the most popular- and useful oils- as well as tools for sharing and the diffuser.

1. The **Premium Starter Kit** contains 11 oils- 5 singles and 6 blends.

- **Single are extracted from one plant- hence, the term "single."**
- **Blends contain multiple oils mixed together, as some of them work well together, amplifying and enhancing the effects of the other.** For these blends, the sum is greater than the parts.

2. The **Starter Kit** contains a few other items, as well.

- **First, let me tell you about our "red drink."** The Premium Starter Kit comes with 2 servings of it, and it's called NingXia Red. NingXia is the name of the province in China where the wolf berry is grown and harvested for this wonderful red drink! The beloved Ningxia Red drink is loaded with antioxidants which help rebuild worn-down cells. And, it's comprised of superfoods that supply your body with the energy it needs for optimal function. Jennifer M. says, "No more afternoon slumps, thanks to NingXia! If for some reason I miss taking it in the morning, I know it by 2pm!"

- **Second, Young Living provides you with a few items to share with your friends.** No hoarding! You can't keep a good thing all to yourself, alright!?

  - *Essential Oils magazine* gives you fun recipes, heart-warming stories and great facts about oils!

  - *Sample bottles and sample sachets* are perfect for "on the go" applications for you- and for sharing with your friends!

  - *Product cards* will give them all the info on what you're sharing with them. Consider them "essential oil cheat" sheets loaded with facts and figures that will keep you one step ahead of everyone else, making you the "go to" person for natural wellness!

- **Third... Young Living includes an $80 valued diffuser in the Premium Starter Kit! Putting a few drops of your favorite essential oil in your diffuser can change the atmosphere of an entire room!** When Cristy received hers, she would give two of her rowdy boys a "time out" in front of the diffuser, instructing them to breathe deeply of the relaxing mist created by just a few drops of lavender oil in the diffuser. (We're not sure if this was for them- or for her- or for both!).

C. The ___twelve___ oils of ancient ___Scripture___.

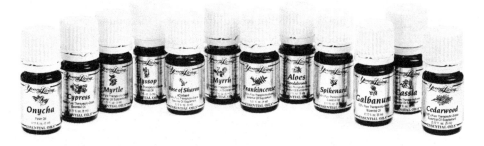

Above: the 12 Oils of Ancient Scripture- we'll walk through these in alphabetical order over the next few pages! We suggest you begin with the Premium Starter Kit and then acquire the 12 Oils of Ancient Scripture. We discuss this in more detail in the appendix ("Start Your Own").

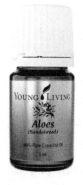

Aloes / Sandalwood is an oil of love. Nicodemus took Sandalwood to prepare Jesus's body for burial, along with Myrrh (John 19:39). David writes of garments being scented with Sandalwood, making one glad (Psalm 45:8).

Some people suggest Sandalwood supports the immune system and the lymphatic system (the lymphatic system is the circulatory system, which is vital to the immune system).

Others suggest Sandalwood serves as an natural aphrodisiac- that it works as a great cologne for men or a natural support for the female reproductive system.

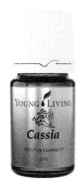

Cassia supports the immune system. Moses included this as an ingredient in the anointing oil for the priests (Exodus 30:22f.). This makes sense when we remember the priests would have handled animal sacrifice daily- and, hence, would have been exposed to their blood any uncleanness or disease they carried.

Also believed to be an anti-fungal, Cassia exudes uplifting feelings. In other words, it's believed that you emotionally feel the effects of the immune support.

We see this cleansing oil mentioned over 50 times throughout the Bible.

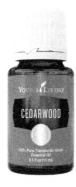

Cedarwood oil addresses the needs of the mind. The wooden beams in the temple were of this tree (1 Kings 4:33, Psalm 104:16). Mentioned 25-plus times throughout the Bible, Cedarwood supports clear thinking.

People have used Cedarwood to address symptoms of ADHD & ADD, as well as hair loss and sleep deprivation.

This oil stimulates the mind in a positive way, and is believed to also facilitate emotional cleansing and release.

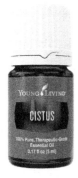

Cistus denotes peace, rest, and refuge. This oil comes from a large white flower found in the fertile plains between Jaffa and Mount Carmel in Israel (sometimes referred to as the Rose of Sharon). In other words, amidst the backdrop of a desert, it is an oasis.

Cistus may promote emotional health and bring a sense of emotional stability. As well, it may also promote physical stability throughout the body; people have been known to use Cistus to ease tremors and / or arthritis pains.

Solomon's wife proclaimed that she was his Rose of Sharon (Song of Solomon 2:1). She was his refuge, his oasis.

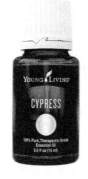

Cypress, in Greek, means "live forever." We learn from the Old Testament that the Temple featured Cypress in addition to Cedarwood (1 Kings 9:11).

The wood is strong and durable- the doors of St. Peter's Cathedral are constructed of Cypress and have been standing unblemished, with no signs of aging, for 1200 years. Perhaps this is why God instructed Noah to build the Ark from Cypress. Tradition says the Cross was Cypress, too, creating eternal salvation in the same way Noah's Ark facilitated temporal salvation.

Cypress may improve circulation, strengthen blood capillaries, and energize white blood cells.

Cypress may be diffused to ease feelings of loss, as well as bring a sense of accompanying emotional ease. In the Temple, Cedarwood assisted the head, while Cypress supported the heart!

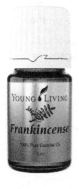

Perhaps the greatest use of Frankincense is spiritual alertness! Extracted from the Boswellia tree, the Biblical word "incense" is translated as *Frankincense*. So, many times when we read *incense* the author is likely referring to this oil.

Frankincense was used to anoint newborn sons of kings throughout the ancient world. The Egyptians believed it was good for "everything from gout to a broken head" (literally, "everything from head to toe"). This explains why many healers in Jesus' day would carry Frankincense with them.

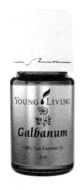

Galbanum exudes grace. In the same way that Jesus declared "I did not come to call the righteous, but sinners..." (Mark 2:17), Galbanum is an oil noted for its ability to address things that are broken or out of balance and bring restoration...

Galbanum has been known to address cramps, abscesses, indigestion, aches & pains, scars, and wrinkles. Galbanum also elevates the mood and helps a person feel whole and alive.

Perhaps this is why Galbum, as part of the Oil of Incense, was diffused in the Temple during the time of sacrifice. People would see- *and sense-* grace in action.

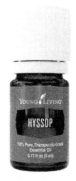

Hyssop means "Holy herb" in Hebrew. Holy means, "set aside for God's use."

Hyssop was believed to erase feelings of guilt and anxiety and bring about a feeling of one-ness with God. This is why David prayed to be cleansed with Hyssop after committing adultery and murder (Psalm 51:7).

Ancients also believed Hyssop could ward off evil spirits, horrible thoughts, and sinful feelings. Remember, the blood of the Passover lamb was smeared with Hyssop on the doorposts (Exodus 12:22), and Jesus was offered a drink while on the Cross with a Hyssop branch (John 19:29).

Hyssop was used to purify temples in the ancient world. This is amazing, considering the Scripture says you are now God's temple (1 Corinthians 6:19).

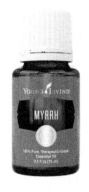

Myrrh was prized for its ability to support healthy skin.
Ancients believed Myrrh helped the skin elude infections, that
it helped reverse stretch marks after birth, and that it was
emotionally uplifting at the same time. If Mary applied Myrrh
to her skin, it would have soothed and calmed baby Jesus
even while supporting her body.

Esther treated her body with Myrrh for 6 months in
preparation for her night with the king (Esther 2:12). Including
her story, we see Myrrh over 150 times in the Bible.

We see Myrrh in the Holy Incense (see Exodus 30:23,34). As
"fixative" Myrrh helps other oils maintain their effects longer
and stronger- which would help since the incense burned 24
hours a day.

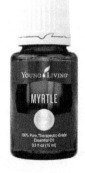

Myrtle is known for supporting the respiratory system- the
throat, the lungs, the nose…

Singers in Solomon's temple are believed to have anointed
their throats with Myrtle. Physicians now believe this would
clear their vocal chords of mucus and allow for better air flow.

Incidentally, Esther's name is Myrtle (*Hadassah*), as her name
was changed in the harem.

Isaiah 55:13 tells us that instead of thorns, Myrtle will grow.
Instead of being choked out, God's people will be able to
spiritually- and physically- breathe!

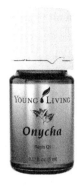

Onycha is a healing oil. Part of the anointing oil referenced in Exodus 30:34, Onycha was used to address open wounds, it was rubbed on the stomach to ease pains, and it was used to stimulate the senses.

This is a thicker oil that almost feels like a gel.

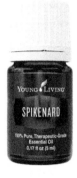

Spikenard reduces nervous tension and soothes. This is the oil used to anoint Jesus- at the beginning of His ministry and just before He faced the Cross (see John 12:3f. and Matthew 26:7f.). The oil reduces anxiety, eases feelings of nausea, and dissolves nervous tension.

Song of Solomon speaks of the table at his home smelling like Spikenard (1:12). Indeed, this oil was prized in the ancient world- remember the objection Judas had to the anointing was that the cost of the oil amounted to a year's wages!

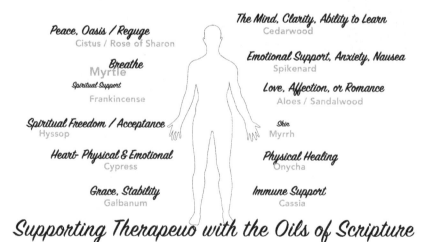

Peace, Oasis / Refuge
Cistus / Rose of Sharon

Breathe
Myrtle

Spiritual Support
Frankincense

Spiritual Freedom / Acceptance
Hyssop

Heart- Physical & Emotional
Cypress

Grace, Stability
Galbanum

The Mind, Clarity, Ability to Learn
Cedarwood

Emotional Support, Anxiety, Nausea
Spikenard

Love, Affection, or Romance
Aloes / Sandalwood

Skin
Myrrh

Physical Healing
Onycha

Immune Support
Cassia

Supporting Therapeuo with the Oils of Scripture

1. Notice how the ___entire___ ___person___ is supported.

- Oils address the physical, emotional, and spiritual needs of the total person.

- God is concerned, then, with the entire person- *body, soul, and spirit.*

2. Did the priests know ___reflexology___? Perhaps they knew more than what we __thought__.

- "Reflexology is an alternative medicine involving application of pressure to the feet and hands with specific thumb, finger, and hand techniques without the use of oil or lotion. It is based on a system of zones and reflex areas that purportedly reflect an image of the body on the feet and hands, with the premise that such work effects a physical change to the body."[134]

- Practitioners of natural healing believe various points on your feet correlate with places on your spine and places throughout your body; they suggest that when you were an embryo, your were "balled up." Gradually, you unfolded and stretched in your mother's womb, developing limbs and organs. However, the connection between those points which were once "one" (i.e., places on your feet, your spine, and various organs in your body) remains!

> OILS ADDRESS THE PHYSICAL, EMOTIONAL, AND SPIRITUAL NEEDS OF THE TOTAL PERSON.

- Therefore, oils touching a place on your body may help in two ways:

[134] Source: https://en.wikipedia.org/wiki/Reflexology, accessed May 3, 2016.

- First, they travel quickly throughout the body- as we discussed earlier.

- Second, every place on your body has unique connections with other places of your body.

- **Compare the ordination of the priests (Leviticus 8) and then consider how God was healing the total man before he ministered healing to the people:**[135]

  - *The ear-* releases and resolves issues regarding their parents.

  - *The thumb-* addresses the fear of the unknown, as well as mental blocks to learning.

  - *The big toe-* deals with addictions and compulsive behavior.[136]

- **Notice, too, that the same protocol for the priests was also followed for the lepers when they were being cleansed** (see Leviticus 14:15-18 NKJV).[137]

---

[135] "Also he took some of its blood and put it on the tip of Aaron's right ear, on the thumb of his right hand, and on the big toe of his right foot. Then he brought Aaron's sons. And Moses put some of the blood on the tips of their right ears, on the thumbs of their right hands, and on the big toes of their right feet" (Leviticus 8:23-24 NKJV).

[136] *Healing Oils of the Bible*, p206.

[137] "15 And the priest shall take some of the log of oil, and pour it into the palm of his own left hand. 16 Then the priest shall dip his right finger in the oil that is in his left hand, and shall sprinkle some of the oil with his finger seven times before the Lord. 17 And of the rest of the oil in his hand, the priest shall put some on the tip of the right ear of him who is to be cleansed, on the thumb of his right hand, and on the big toe of his right foot, on the blood of the trespass offering. 18 The rest of the oil that is in the priest's hand he shall put on the head of him who is to be cleansed. So the priest shall make atonement for him before the Lord" (Leviticus 14:15-18 NKJV).

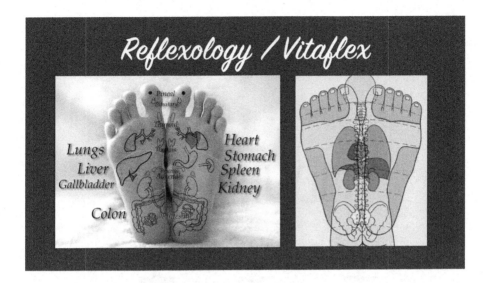

On the left, reflexology for the feet. On the right, an easier-to-understand diagram showing the placement of the various organs throughout the body. Don't think you can memorize the entire chart? Just anoint the entire foot and everything is covered.

This raises an interesting question: Is there more to foot washing than we might have thought? Is foot washing something that not only cleansed a weary traveler physically, but also created an environment of intimacy and healing?

3. Once you understand the __basics__ of the __oils__, you'll probably begin recognizing them throughout the __Bible__.

- **There are a few places we see the Oils of the Scripture *together*.** Let's look at a few of those examples. You may study others on your own.

- For our purposes in this workbook we'll look at the Holy Incense (Exodus 30:34-36), the protocol for cleaning the lepers (Leviticus 14), and Jesus' birth.

HOLY INCENSE

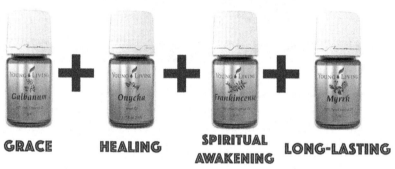

GRACE   HEALING   SPIRITUAL AWAKENING   LONG-LASTING

Notice how each of these oils "fit" together to make a perfect blend for the Temple. First, we see grace in action (Galbanum). And, we see the presence of healing (Onycha), along with spiritual awakening (Frankincense). This sounds a lot like sozo, the third word for healing we learned earlier. As well, Myrrh elevates and magnifies the qualities of all other oils, and is noted for its ability to bring peace and calm- to the body, soul, and spirit.

Remember, today, you are the temple (1 Corinthians 6:19). This is the same power-combo that resides in you- Grace, Healing, Spiritual Awakening, and Long-lasting Peace.

CLEANSING LEPERS

CLARITY OF MIND

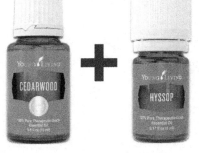

CLEANSED OF GUILT & SHAME

Notice two of the oils used to anoint lepers. We see they were given a renewed mind (Cedarwood), which would see reality differently. And, they were cleansed of the old guilt and shame associated with their disease (Hyssop). Many New Testament scholars believe leprosy is a "type" (read: foreshadowing) of sin- as sin separates us from others, it brings its unique stigma and condemnation, and it becomes our identity. However, we are given a renewed mind (Romans 12:1-2) and we are cleansed wholly!

JESUS' BIRTH

**SPIRITUAL /
SON OF
A KING**

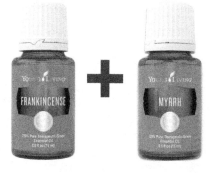

**SOOTHING-
BODY,
EMOTIONS, &
SPIRIT**

The birth of Jesus is highlighted by the unique gifts the magi brought to Him. One was the same oil used to anoint all newborn sons of kings in the ancient world- and was the "go to" for healing (Frankincense). The other brings peace and comfort to the body, soul, and spirit (Myrrh). Is this not what Jesus came to do?

Apply Habit 2 & Anoint

WHAT DO YOU NEED?
THE OILS OF THE PREMIUM STARTER KIT
THE TWELVE OILS OF ANCIENT SCRIPTURE

☐ I love this verse from 1 Corinthians 3:22-23. That church was apparently arguing over which teacher was better. In response, Paul told them that "all things are yours: whether Paul or Apollos or Cephas…"That is, they didn't have to pick a teacher; they could take the best from all of them. He continues, though, explaining just how many things are theirs. He says, "…or the world or life or death, or things present or things to come—all are yours. And you are Christ's, and Christ is God's." The words he uses are the same words we use to denote biology, including how life works and how death happens. He tells the church, in effect, "Everything here is yours… Everything." How does this relate to health and wellness, to *therapeuo*?

☐ The oils are simply tools God uses. The power of healing still comes from the Father. How can you articulate this to others in such a way that they don't feel like you've turned into a "voodoo witch doctor" with lotions and potions?

☐ Paul wrote to Timothy, "For everything God created is good, and nothing is to be rejected if it is received with thanksgiving" (1 Timothy 4:4). Of course, this assumption is that "it is sanctified by the word of God and prayer" (4:5). Tell me what you learn from this verse as it relates to *therapeuo*?

☐ We discussed supporting the "total person"- body, soul, and spirit. Do you see anything new from this chapter that you've not been exposed to before? In what ways does supporting the total person fit with *sozo*? Can some *sozo* be experienced by *therapeuo*?

☐ What do you make about the similarity between the ordination of the priests (Leviticus 8:1f.) and the healing protocol for lepers (Leviticus 14:15f.)?

☐ What do you see about the different ways the oils are used? Did you identify specific oils which may be helpful to you?

Oils I'd Like to Try

ISSUE	OIL I'D LIKE TO TRY

☐ Is this list above broader than you thought it might be at first?

☐ What other oils do you think would be useful to have?

APPLY HABIT 2 & ANOINT

- _____
- _____
- _____
- _____
- _____

☐ Do you have your oils yet? If not, see the "Start Your Own" section in the appendix for info on how to obtain them.

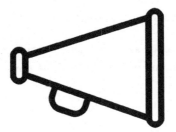

5. Habit 3 = Tell

TOUCH THE BODY, SOUL, & SPIRIT
YOU CARRY THE PRESENCE & POWER
FOCUS ON WHAT'S RIGHT

"Faith comes by hearing" (Romans 10:17).

"He sent His word and healed them" (Psalm 107:20).

"Life and death are in the power of the tongue" (Proverbs 18:21).

A. Touch the __body__, __soul__, and __spirit__.

- The Father is interested in your *total* healing- and in the *complete* healing of the people around you.

- As we've already seen, many times the core issues are healed first (i.e., identity, unforgiveness) and the physical issues follow...

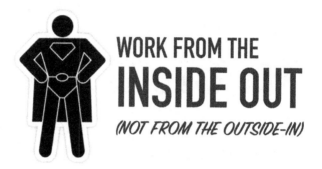

WORK FROM THE
INSIDE OUT
(NOT FROM THE OUTSIDE-IN)

1. You are primarily a ___**spirit**with a ___**body**. Our assumption, then, when seeking healing is that the __**deepest**__ issues are there. We want to work from the "__**inside**__ **out**__," from the core, addressing the total person.

- It wasn't until the 20th Century that physical healing and spiritual healing were separated.

- Remember, in the Old Testament people with physical issues were sent to the priests; in the New Testament people were sent to the elders of the church.

> IN ORDER FOR TRUE HEALING TO MANIFEST, WE MUST ADDRESS THE WHOLE PERSON.

- **Allopathic forms of care do not heal the entire person.** They have a tremendous place, but they only focus on the body.[138] And, generally, allopathic protocols are reactive (fix)- not proactive (prevent).

  - In order for true healing to manifest, we must address the whole person.

  - Remember, the limbic system stores harmful and hurtful memories throughout the body- where they often manifest as physical issues. In a real sense, these physical ailments, then, are simply symptoms of an emotional or spiritual hurt. If we don't address the deeper issue, we're simply covering the "check engine light" as we discussed earlier

ALLOPATHIC	THERAPEUO
Fix	Prevent
Body	Body, Soul, Spirit

---

[138] From wikipedia.com, accessed April 12, 2016: "Allopathic medicine is an expression commonly used by homeopaths and proponents of other forms of alternative medicine to refer to mainstream medical use of pharmacologically active agents or physical interventions to treat or suppress symptoms or pathophysiologic processes of diseases or conditions.[1] The expression was coined in 1810 by the creator of homeopathy, Samuel Hahnemann (1755–1843).[2] In such circles, the expression "allopathic medicine" is still used to refer to "the broad category of medical practice that is sometimes called Western medicine, biomedicine, evidence-based medicine, or modern medicine" (see the article on scientific medicine).

2. As the __spirit__ finds healing, the _body_ quickly moves into alignment.

B. You carry the _presence_ and _power_ of the Kingdom.

1. Jesus' measures of the Kingdom seem _different_ than ours.

- **We read Him saying things that indicate that the Kingdom is accompanied by power- and that the Kingdom is present:**

    - "... announce and preach the Kingdom of God... bring healing" (Luke 9:2 AMP).

    - "heal the sick... say to them, 'The Kingdom of God has come close to you'" (Luke 10:9 AMP).

> JESUS' MEASURE OF THE KINGDOM WAS BASED ON PEOPLE ENCOUNTERING THE PRESENCE OF THE FUTURE NOW.

    - "The kingdom of God does not come with your careful observation, nor will people say, 'Here it is,' or 'There it is,' because the kingdom of God is within you" (Luke 17:20-21).

- In other words, **Jesus' measure of the Kingdom was based on people encountering the presence of the future *now*.** The presence of the Kingdom was- and is- the presence of Heaven invading this moment. When that happens, healing comes.

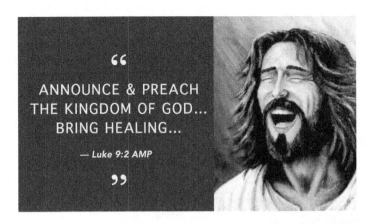

> " ANNOUNCE & PREACH THE KINGDOM OF GOD... BRING HEALING...
> — *Luke 9:2 AMP*
> "

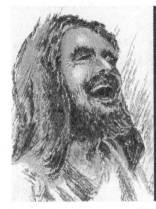

> " HEAL THE SICK... SAY TO THEM, "THE KINGDOM OF GOD HAS COME CLOSE TO YOU!"
> — *Luke 10:9 AMP*
> "

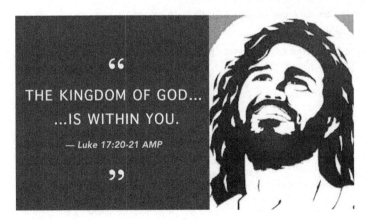

> " THE KINGDOM OF GOD... ...IS WITHIN YOU.
> — *Luke 17:20-21 AMP*
> "

2. Our measures most often revolve around __nickels__ & __noses___ (How many people were in the __seats_? How much __money_ did they __give_?).

- **We've shifted from the idea of a planting a peaceful Kingdom that infuses all of life to the strategy of simply planting church services.** Every metric we use to evaluate our success as a church is reduced to how many people occupy seats during a weekly gathering- and how many of those people gave some money to the ministry.[139]

- **Don't get me wrong- I'm *pro*-church!** I'm in favor of worship services. I encounter the Lord at them. I'm inspired when I see others encountering Him. I learn. I'm stretched. I'm encouraged when I see a larger group of people and am reminded that we are on the same page, that we're "in this together."

- **However, those meetings are not the sum total of the Kingdom- even though we often reduce the sum total of evaluating the Kingdom to how those services are going.**[140] We measure noses and nickels. How many people were there? How many money did they give? Sometimes we even measure raised hands, as if a raised hand while no one is looking (everyone has to bow their head and close their eyes, usually, per the preacher's instructions to give people privacy while they may a public confession) in any way indicates that we have a joined a revolutionary movement of bringing Heaven present to earth.

---

[139] Now that we've maxed out our facilities, we've created "online" campuses that we count as part of our numbers. I'm obviously a proponent of online media, but...

[140] I don't know a single pastor would say this is the sum total of the kingdom- to be honest. At the same time, I only know a few who measure other things besides nickels and noses.

3. What if our measures were more like ___*Christ's*___?

- **What if we measured helping people encounter the Presence and taking that Presence with them when they left the building?** What if we carried the *iaomai* and *therapeuo* that Jesus spoke about- and empowered His disciples to take- with us?

- **What if we measured the full scope of salvation-** of people who were rescued from addictions, people who were physically healed of something terminal, people who were delivered from oppression (spiritual and physical)? In other words, *sozo.*

> WHAT IF OUR MEASURES WERE MORE LIKE CHRIST'S?

- **What if we measured how effective we were at releasing people into ministry-** not into serving our system of necessary parking lot attendants, ushers and greeters, and other "slots" that keep our machine running- but truly into doing what they were called to do?[141]

- **What if we lived life in such community that we didn't only measure life change during the snap shot of an "invitation / response time" at a church service, but we walked with people long term?** What if we knew their stories and saw the ripple of effect through their life for 3 years? 10 years? Through the next generation?

- **What if we tangibly measured the effect of the church on our city?** Is homelessness down because the church is present? Are marriages in our city stronger because the church is here? Is the economy better because the church is alive?[142] Even in the Old Testament these were indicators that God used to show the people that He was among

---

[141] Again, I'm grateful for people who serve in these areas. They're needed. But Jesus empowered us to make disciples (Matthew 28:18-20) and lay hands on the sick (Mark 16:15f.).

[142] Yes, the economy. In the Old Testament, God promised to bless His people- and even give them the power to get wealth (see Deuteronomy 8:18, for instance).

them.[143] If the New Testament is a better covenant (which I believe it to be), then wouldn't these indicators work, too? You see, God refuses to let us live lives that persist as if His Word is merely "spiritual" and doesn't bring "physical" results.

4. The reality is this: when people encounter _you_ they actually encounter __everything_ of the Kingdom.

- **Jesus empowers us in the same way the Father empowered Him.**

  - Jesus said that whenever people saw Him they actually saw the Father. He revealed the Father completely (John 14:7-9). We discussed this in chapter 1, when we talked about believing the right things about God as a foundational touchpoint for a healing ministry.[144]

  - He also said that He sends us in the same way that He was sent: "As the Father sent me, I send you" (John 20:21). To me, this doesn't just mean that "The Father sent Him and He is sending us." Rather, it means "He is sending us *in the same manner* that the Father sent Him."

> WE READ THAT THE FULLNESS OF THE DEITY DWELLED IN JESUS... WE ALSO READ THAT JESUS IS IN US- WITH HIS FULLNESS...

  - We read that the fullness of the deity dwelled in Jesus (Colossians 1:19).

  - We also read that Jesus is in us- with His fullness (Colossians 1:27).

---

[143] See Isaiah 65:17, for instance. We know he's writing about the present- not Heaven- because we see the presence of sin and death (65:20), things which don't exist in Heaven. See also Isaiah 55.

[144] Yes, now we're coming back "full circle" to where we began this book.

- It's easy to see, then, that we become an encounter, a connector to the Presence and Power of Christ and all of our Father's Kingdom. *How could we not with everything that He has resourced to us?*

- **This is, perhaps, what Paul meant when He wrote about the life of Christ in the believer.**

  - "For me to *live is Christ...*" (Philippians 1:21)

  - "I... no longer live... *Christ lives in me...*" (Galatians 2:20)

- **In other words, you are the *same* as Christ on this earth...**

  - "As He is, so are we..." (1 John 4:17)

  - Think about *light. We are told to walk in the light, as He is Light (see 1 John 1:7)*

    - We read this multiple times in the New Testament- Jesus is Light (see also John 1:7). He even said Himself, "I am the Light of the world" (John 8:12).

    - In like manner, we read that *you* are light (see Ephesians 5:8). In fact, Jesus Himself declared it: "You are the light of the world" (Matthew 5:14).

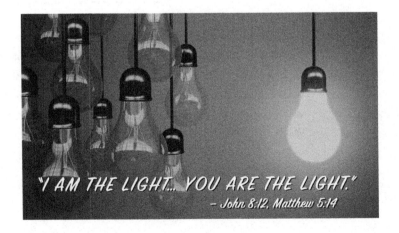

"I AM THE LIGHT... YOU ARE THE LIGHT."
— John 8:12, Matthew 5:14

You Are An Encounter...

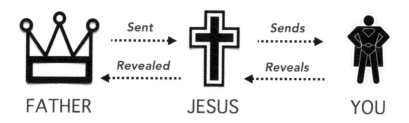

| FATHER | JESUS | YOU |

- You were created in His image and likeness (Genesis 1:26-27). What part of this has the Cross and Resurrection not resolved?

- **To encounter you is to encounter Him.** Because of the Cross, the old nature is gone and you have a new nature- His nature. In fact, the Bible tells us that you live His very life... or, that He lives that life through you.[145]

> YOU WERE CREATED IN HIS IMAGE AND LIKENESS (GENESIS 1:26-27). WHAT PART OF THIS HAS THE CROSS AND RESURRECTION NOT RESOLVED?

- This idea that *you are an encounter* plays out in the story of the Woman at the Well / The Samaritan Woman (John 4:1f.). After asking her for a drink, Jesus suggests to her that she would have asked Him for a drink if she knew who He really was. He then tells her that whoever takes a drink of the Living Water that He gives will...

---

[145] See the *Grace Basics* video series. It's part of the online version of this class- and is included in the bonus materials. Video 6, "You are an encounter" goes into more detail on this point. For more info: www.GraceBasics.info.

- Never thirst again (4:10). They will be satisfied (meaning you will be satisfied instead of empty or dry). *And,*

- They will have a spring of water welling up, which Jesus provides to them, that comes from within (4:10). That is, they will be become a *source*- an encounter of that same water.

  - *Not a well.* Wells aren't sources. They tap *into* a source and give you access to it. They are merely conduits.

  - *Not a cistern.* Cisterns are simply containers. You put water in them to store for later use. They aren't even tied to a source. They are simply holding tanks.

  - *A spring.* Jesus says that you will be a spring of living water- that you will be a *source*. Not that you will be tied to a source- but that you will actually be a source. You will be an encounter.[146]

3 Sources of Water...

WELL MUST BE CONNECTED TO A SOURCE

CISTERN MUST BE RE-FILLED, IS ONLY A CONTAINER

SPRING IS A SOURCE!

---

[146] In other words, many people are looking externally for something they already carry. The Kingdom is *within* you. Already. See Luke 17:21.

C. Focus on what's ___*right*___, and move above the wellness line!

1. At least seven things can raise your ___*frequency*___ to a __*higher*__ level.

1. **First, studies have shown that your thoughts can raise and lower your frequencies**, too- by as much as 10 MHz in either direction![147]

   - Proverbs 23:7 says, "As a man thinks, so is he…"

   - Of course, this fits with Habit 1 (Think). [148]

   - In addition, Quantum Physics is confirming that the way in which the world around us expresses itself to us has more to do with what we expect to see than any other factor! For instance, "Whether energy expresses itself as a wave or a particle seems to be related to the expectation of the observer. In Quantum Physics experiments, if the observer is expecting to see waves, the energy behaves as waves. If the observer is expecting to see particles, the energy behaves as particles."[149]

---

[147] *Healing Oils of the Bible*, p33.

[148] From chapter 6, "Good Vibrations" in *The Physics of Heaven*, p63 (Ellyn Davis): "We've also had incidents of synchronicity such as thinking of a person and suddenly having them call us. Many scientists are convinced these experiments indicate that thoughts and emotions, as well as words, carry vibrational frequencies that radiate into our surroundings and not only affect our own thoughts and emotions but also affect everything and everyone around us. However, no instrumentation has yet been developed to measure the vibrational frequencies of thoughts or emotions."

[149] See p112 in chapter 11, "Strange Things are Afoot," from *The Physics of Heaven*, Ellyn Davis and Judy Franklin.

- Ever had a day where everything went your way simply because you expected it to? Or even the opposite- everything went as bad as you thought it would!

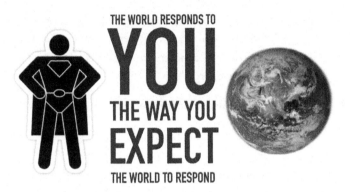

THE WORLD RESPONDS TO **YOU** THE WAY YOU **EXPECT** THE WORLD TO RESPOND

2. Second, emotions can raise your frequency. Or lower them.

- Proverbs 17:22 tells us that "a merry heart does good like a medicine."

- On the flip side, we see that negative emotions are harmful. Consider Proverbs 14:30: "A sound mind makes for a robust body, but runaway emotions corrode the bones" (MSG).

- Does this *really* have anything to do with your health and healing? Probably more than you think. Consider what bone marrow actually does: "…bone marrow produces approximately 500 billion blood cells per day, which use the bone marrow vasculature as a conduit to the body's systemic circulation. Bone marrow is also a key component of the lymphatic system, producing the lymphocytes that support the body's immune system."[150]

---

[150] Source: https://en.wikipedia.org/wiki/Bone_marrow, accessed 05/11/2016.

- "… everything- even our thoughts and emotions- emits energetic vibrations…" As odd as this may sound at first glance, "many people believe this without attributing it to Quantum Physics because we've all had experiences such as sensing the tension when we walk into a room where people have been arguing. Metaphyisicsts would say we are picking up on the 'vibrations' of anger… Some vibrations are good and give off healing energy… others give off damaging, unhealthy energy."[151]

3. **Third, touch can raise your frequency.**

    - We discussed the healing power of physical touch earlier in the books. And, though this is area we might tend to overlook we should embrace it- especially in our disconnected world. *Touch matters.*[152]

    > YOUR BODY, WHEN HEALTHY, IS FIGHTING FOR HEALTH- NOT FIGHTING FOR DISEASE.

    - "Dr. Walter Weston reports in *Prayer Heals* that most people emit a variable electromagnetic frequency from their hands, but healers emit a steady 7.8 hertz frequency… Researchers shown that the hands of spiritual healers can emit over 200 volts of electricity whereas non-healers' hands produce no more than 4 volts. 200 volts is more than the voltage used in electrocardioversion to reset heart rhythm."[153]

4. **Fourth, the oils can raise your frequency.** We discussed this in great detail in the final section of Habit 2 (Touch).

---

[151] See chapter 12, "Quantum Mysticism," by Ellyn Davis in *The Physics of Heaven*. This quote comes from pp124-125.

[152] See earlier where we discussed the healing power of physical touch.

[153] Quoted from p29 of *The Physics of Heaven*.

5. **Fifth, sound can raise your frequency.** The words we say (and listen to), as well as the music we choose, matters.

- "Sound can create a story from dry facts. It causes our emotions to go beyond facts to feelings... The revelation that comes to the seer has everything to do with *the sound* of the scene being viewed."[154]

- Consider movie soundtracks. If you see a person running frantically down the street in the middle of the night, you'll instantly feel different about what is happening if you hear the screeching theme to *Psycho* playing in the background as opposed to Rocky's *Eye of the Tiger.*

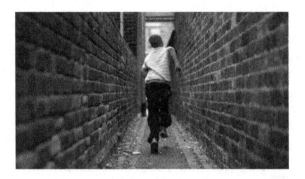

6. **Sixth, prayer can raise your frequency.**

- Prayer makes an even greater change than positive thoughts, notching someone's frequency up by 15 MHz![155]

- Think about the difference prayer can make with oils and with positive confession! Imagine what happens with them together!

---

[154] See chapter 7, "Sound of Heaven / Symphony of Earth," in *The Physics of Heaven.* Ray Hughes is the author of the chapter. See p69. Emphasis added.

[155] *Healing Oils of the Bible,* p33.

- "Prayer can work without the oils. Oils can work without prayer… If you are having success with prayer along, it can be increased by the intelligent use of oils. If you are having success with oils, apply them with prayer and you will see even greater success."[156]

7. **Seventh, healthy food raises your frequency** (also reviewed in Habit 2). Your physical and spiritual breakthrough may very well include the foods you choose to eat. Remember, a lifestyle of *therapeuo* is one of the forms of faith that is backed by action!

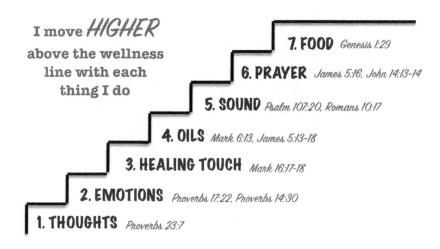

I move *HIGHER* above the wellness line with each thing I do

7. FOOD *Genesis 1:29*

6. PRAYER *James 5:16, John 14:13-14*

5. SOUND *Psalm 107:20, Romans 10:17*

4. OILS *Mark 6:13, James 5:13-18*

3. HEALING TOUCH *Mark 16:17-18*

2. EMOTIONS *Proverbs 17:22, Proverbs 14:30*

1. THOUGHTS *Proverbs 23:7*

Is there a certain order to all of this? Not necessarily. Many of these areas actually overlap. When you pray (7), for instance, you flood the atmosphere with a positive sound (5) that stirs the thoughts (1) and emotions (2). The oils (4) reach the emotions (2), also, because of the limbic system. Eating better (7) also causes you to feel better (2) and think more positively about yourself (1). They all work together… and they all move you higher above the wellness line.

---

[156] *Healing Oils of the Bible*, p93.

2. The best environment for __*healing*__ simply takes advantage of __*everything*___ God has created.

- **A perfect scenario for bringing healing in your household, I believe, is the following:**

    - Walk in a lifestyle of *therapeuo*, of health and healing (including diet and exercise, avoiding toxins and supplementing as necessary).

    - Use the oils regularly for general needs and specifically when they are needed for a particular cause.

    - Speak a positive confession as to what is going to happen, declaring the *iaomai* and *sozo* Christ has provided. Remember, often end up seeing manifest exactly what we wanted to see![157]

    - Release the healing power of touch to your family, friends, and those to whom you minister healing.

    - Pray and thank God, declaring reality to be true on earth as it is in Heaven.

- **Understand, your natural state is health and wholeness.** Your body, when healthy, is fighting for health- not fighting for disease. Your body, when healthy and whole, is moving *higher* in frequency. On a Biblical level, this is because you are created in God's image (Genesis 1:27). He *does not* have disease or illness.[158] And, there is no illness or sickness in Heaven. Jesus says that you live the presence of the Kingdom, now" (Luke 12:32 and Luke 17:21, for instance). As such,

---

[157] See a video about this at www.WeOverflow.com/See.

[158] Some people believe God gives illness and sickness and disease to people. I do not believe this to be the case. We address this in Habit 1: Think.

healing, your naturally-created state as well as your end destination, are available in this present moment.

- The oils simply help "restore the body back to its natural state of balance and health at the most basic and fundamental levels." They may do this instantly (*iaomai*, as we learned in the previous chapter), over time (*therapeuo*), or a combination of both.[159] **Again, healing is your natural state; you were designed to be well- not created to be sick.**

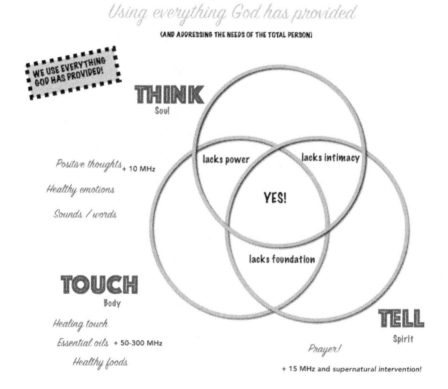

Using everything God has provided

(AND ADDRESSING THE NEEDS OF THE TOTAL PERSON)

WE USE EVERYTHING GOD HAS PROVIDED!

THINK
Soul

Positive thoughts + 10 MHz

Healthy emotions

Sounds / words

lacks power

lacks intimacy

YES!

lacks foundation

TOUCH
Body

Healing touch

Essential oils + 50-300 MHz

Healthy foods

TELL
Spirit

Prayer!

+ 15 MHz and supernatural intervention!

---

[159] *Healing Oils of the Bible*, p31.

3. Focus on __salvation__ (total __SOZO__) and the __Savior__- not sin, not Satan, not something else.

- Earlier in the book I mentioned that some people believe God causes them to be sick. We rejected that notion. **God is the author of health and wellness- *not* death and disease.**

- We discussed how many view faith- that you must have *complete faith* to receive healing. I suggested that wasn't true, either. With so many examples throughout the Bible ranging from bold faith to "no faith," you can't "create a theological box" that's a one-size-fits-all scenario. **Faith is *not* a "work" we must do in order to merit health and wellness.**

- The same is true when evaluating the conditions causing the need for healing prayer. **There are numerous reasons we- or someone we know- may find themselves unwell.** (Here, be aware that you do *not* necessarily

> HEALING IS YOUR NATURAL STATE; YOU WERE DESIGNED TO BE WELL- NOT CREATED TO BE SICK.

  need to verbally communicate everything you discern.)[160] You can simply pray and release the Kingdom's power. Here's what I mean. There are *three* general reasons someone may need healing:

  1. ***Sin can cause unwellness.*** Yes, sin can cause illness. Or harm. Sometimes it is our own sin; other times it is others' sins against us (as in the case of abuse, a drunk driver who crashes into someone, etc.). It's important to remember that God isn't "getting us" for chastising us for doing something wrong by

---

[160] Sometimes, God gives you insight so you know how to better love the person- not berate, embarrass, or condemn them. Always honor the people before you. This means you do not necessarily need to say everything He reveals to you. Part of knowing what to say and what not to say involves both wisdom and practical experience.

inflicting us with illness; most often, these are instances of simply reaping what we sow.[161]

- I have seen instances of reaping the rotten fruit of sowing bad health habits. For instance:

  - My granddaddy died of lung cancer. It wasn't because God was judging him; God already judged Jesus on my granddaddy's behalf on the Cross. My granddaddy died of lung cancer because he chain-smoked for years. Even decades.

  - When I was working at churches and nonprofit ministries, I had staff members who've faced various health issues. God wasn't judging them. In fact, I believe He's incredibly happy with the turnaround they've made. They've walked out of an old life, into a new one, and are now helping others make that transition. But, they carry some scars from the old life. It's not His judgment for bad choices in the past; it's reaping what was sown in those years. Miraculously, we saw most of them healed![162]

> MOST OFTEN, THESE ARE INSTANCES OF SIMPLY REAPING WHAT WE SOW.

---

[161] Sow unwellness and you will reap unwellness. Remember, *therapeuo* almost always involves lifestyle change and new habits.

[162] And, keeping true to the pattern we see in this book, *iaomai* came for some- then they stewarded the healing by walking in *therapeuo*. Others walked *therapeuo*, persisting for the miracle with patience- even as they got better through their lifestyle changes.!

- We see this in the Bible:

  - Jesus healed the man at the Pool of Bethesda (a man who had no idea who Jesus was, by the way, thereby showing us something important about the faith issue). Jesus later runs into the man (who, again, doesn't even know who Jesus is), telling him "go and sin no more, lest something worse happen to you" (worse than a 38-year illness!) (see 5:14). Jesus apparently linked the sickness to the sin in this situation, though we are not sure how the man sinned to cause this illness. Note, then: sickness (which I'm defining as any situation less than perfect health- physically or emotionally) can result from sin. The sin, though, may not necessarily be someone's fault.[163] For instance, in the cases of rape or abuse, sin may be the direct cause of a condition needing to be addressed. However, *it does not mean that the sin is the fault of the person needing healing.*

  - The disciples realized this as asked Jesus about the man who was born blind (in John 9:1f.) that we will review in a moment: "Who sinned to cause this? The man... or his parents...?" They saw a direct link between sin and sickness- one that Jesus corrected in this instance. Notice, though, Jesus didn't say, "Sin can't cause

---

[163] This is an important distinction. People can be hurt by the sins of others. When this occurs, they are not guilty of the sin- at all. But, they may need cleansing from the effects of the sin. Forgiveness may bring quick release and healing.

unwellness." He simply suggested this wasn't the case in this instance.

- It's important to remember that God has *forgotten* your sin if you are a Christian.[164] As I mentioned earlier, you may reap what you've sown somewhere.

> GOD HAS FORGOTTEN YOUR SIN AND REMOVED THE SIN. HE HAS CLEANSED IT. YOU ARE WHOLE... HE IS NOT GOING TO PUNISH YOU WITH AN ILLNESS.

However, God has forgotten your sin and removed the sin. He has cleansed it. You are whole. As such, you can rest assured He is not going to punish you with an illness.

  - The exception to this is that I've seen unforgiveness actually manifest as an illness. Somehow, it creates a bitter root that births fruit in the form of un-health. I've seen it over and over, that believers often have a bitterness they are holding. When it is released, the healing often happens- even without praying and asking for it.[165]

  - Let me give you a word of extreme caution: Be extremely careful when blaming sin for someone's condition. Even if this is the case, it does not necessarily need to be said- you may simply pastor the person

---

[164] Hebrews 8:12, Hebrews 10:17. See also the *Grace Basics* video number 7, "Giving Sin Too Much Attention." It's including in the bonus materials of the online course.

[165] Again, the limbic system stores harmful memories throughout the body until you are ready to deal with them. Because of this, many physical ailments simply disappear once the memory has been handled (through forgiveness and release), as the body no longer "hangs on."

through the situation, speaking the life-giving message of the Gospel to them, and praying for their total freedom. In other words, don't focus on what caused the issue; focus on the remedy. Don't team up with the side of the accusation; join with restoration.

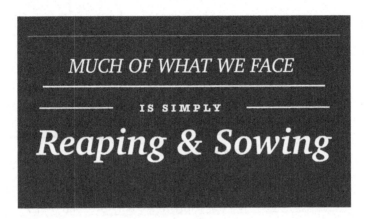

MUCH OF WHAT WE FACE

IS SIMPLY

Reaping & Sowing

2. ***Satan can cause unwellness***. The enemy can taunt people. And does. We see examples of this throughout the New Testament. It's odd to me that many well-intended Christians are hesitant to attribute things to the devil (like cancer) that they will actually ascribe to God ("God gave me this, so...").[166]

   • If you are a follower of Christ, you *can* be harassed by a demon. You can be oppressed, such that it manifests in the form of an illness, depression (which

---

[166] It's odd to me that many people blame God for disease instead of blaming the Devil. Incidentally, many of the same people see poverty as a blessing and abundance as a curse. It seems we may have our theological lines crossed.

is a form of mental illness / mental un-health), and even anxiety. If you are a follower of Christ, you *cannot* be inhabited (read: possessed) by a demon.[167]

- Many Christians believe that because they are in Christ, they cannot be taunted by demons. A Christian *cannot* be inhabited by a demon- the Holy Spirit inhabits a Christian. However, a Christian can be, as Paul was, pestered by them (see 2 Corinthians 12:7, again).[168] Paul says he was "buffeted" by a messenger of Satan, meaning that he was struck repeatedly, over and over. Apparently, he prayed for the Lord to handle it, but was given grace to be perfected in his weakness (12:9), despite three earnest pleas for deliverance (12:8).[169]

> CHRISTIANS ARE HESITANT TO ATTRIBUTE THINGS TO THE DEVIL (LIKE CANCER) THAT THEY WILL ACTUALLY ASCRIBE TO GOD ("GOD GAVE ME THIS, SO...").

- Jesus heals one such woman while He is teaching one Saturday (the Sabbath was Saturday). Here is what we see:

---

[167] The New Testament doesn't actually use the word "possessed." Rather, the word is *demonized*. This actually makes it a bit more difficult to understand what is happening, because the word can refer to *oppression* or *possession*, two different labels we interject to help us understand what is happening.

[168] It is helpful to remember that demons occupy the second realm, whereas you and Christ occupy the third (Ephesians 1:20-2:6). You are above them.

[169] Mother Teresa writes of this same feeling in her memoirs.

- She has been ill for 18 years (Luke 13:11). She cannot stand straight, or even look anyone in the eye (Luke 13:11). She doesn't seek the healing; Jesus sees her, calls out to her, and frees her with a word (Luke 13:12).[170]

- He then laid hands on her, and she was able to stand straight. The affliction in her back was loosened with His touch (Luke 13:12).[171]

- Some translations tells us from the outset that the infirmity was caused by an evil spirit (Luke 13:11). It becomes clearer when we hear Jesus interact with the leaders of the synagogue, all of whom are angered because it is the Sabbath (Luke 13:14).

- He tells them, "Ought not this woman, a daughter of Abraham, whom Satan has bound for eighteen years, be loosed from this bond on the Sabbath day" (Luke 13:16 AMP)? Jesus explains to them that they would assist an animal needing help; therefore, they should be even more willing to help

> THE BIBLE TELLS US THAT ALL THINGS WORK TOGETHER FOR THE GOOD... IT DOES NOT TELL US THAT ALL THINGS ARE GOOD. IT DOES NOT TELL THAT GOD CAUSES ALL THINGS.

---

[170] Notice this dynamic again: Jesus can heal with words alone, but He often touches the people too.

[171] Notice how He uses touch here- as a woman, she would have been considered a "second class" citizen in that culture. And, as someone with an illness, people would have likely supposed she had a sin issue that caused it.

her- particularly since she *is* a daughter of Abraham (Luke 13:15). Again, she is a daughter of Abraham (Luke 13:16), answering the question that people of the faith family can be opposed by Satan, even though not possessed. As such, healing and wholeness are part of her inheritance.

3. *Something else can cause unwellness*. There may be other reasons for unwellness that defy categorization. In other words, this is the "junk drawer" where I simply place any other instance.

    - The Bible tells us that *all* things work together for the good (Romans 8:28). It does not tell us that all things *are* good. It does not tell that God *causes* all things. Rather, it tells us that God causes all things to work for the good. Many things are attributed to God that clearly do not fit His character.

    - Many people are afraid to simply admit they don't have an answer as to why someone needs healing. However, *you need to be comfortable with not supplying an answer when you don't have one*. It's OK to not know the reason why someone is sick- we know Who makes them well! *You don't need the cause; you just need the cure!*

    - The default answer I see most often given in these times is, "It must be God's will..." However, as we've seen, this doesn't fit with His character or the thrust of Scripture.

- **Be mindful when suggesting any of these causes to someone. Again, we want to focus on the cure- not the cause.** And there are multiple reasons why!

- *If you suggest sin is the reason they need healing, they may feel condemned.* This was clearly the case with the lame man who was waiting to get pushed into the Pool at Bethesda. Yet, Jesus never worried that this man's theology wasn't accurate- nor did He correct him of the sin issue before healing him.

- *If you suggest Satan has taunted them, they may be alarmed.* Face it: we do need to place any more focus on him than he's already garnered. When Jesus healed the "daughter of Abraham" who had been tormented for decades, He simply healed her. No rebuking or yelling needed at the enemy was required (Luke 13:10f.).

> IT'S OK TO NOT KNOW THE REASON WHY SOMEONE IS SICK- WE KNOW WHO MAKES THEM WELL! YOU DON'T NEED THE CAUSE; YOU JUST NEED THE CURE!

- *If you suggest God has caused them their distress, they may feel unloved.* And, of course, you would be working against the grain of the New Testament on this one. We spoke about this in chapter 1 when we discussed "Think Right About God."

  - Some say that God causes sickness to bring glory to Himself. The greater glory, though, is when we acknowledge that the provision of Christ was enough, that God Himself in Christ Jesus has made us whole. It doesn't bring me glory as a father when my kids are walking around ill; it brings me honor when they are healthy, happy, and whole. The same is true of our Heavenly Father.

- Others say God causes sickness in order to purify them. This point-of-view too says that the Cross wasn't enough, that somehow we must still walk "through something" in order to complete the process of sanctification (making us holy) that God wants to achieve. People like this often view God more like "The Godfather" than "God the Father."

What Caused the Dis-ease?

IF YOU SUGGEST...	THEY MAY FEEL...
SIN	Condemned
SATAN	Alarmed
SOMETHING ELSE	Confused
GOD	Unloved

4. Assume your ___Father___ is there to ___bless___ people- and focus on this.

- **Notably, in the Old Testament, sickness is always a curse and healing is always a blessing (see Deuteronomy 28, for instance).** In the Old Testament, people were expected to obey and then they would receive that blessing. If not, they would receive the curse. I've yet to find any examples in which sickness is a blessing and health is a curse. Yet, even in the New Testament era, a time period we know is founded on "better promises" than the Old (Hebrews 8:6).[172] And, Jesus has completed our total obedience.[173]

- **It's odd that we've turned the Biblical paradigm around.**[174] In the Bible, good things come from God; and He never adjusts to reveal a dark side (James 1:17).

  - In a real sense, I believe that we've "turned the paradigm around" in order to explain issues for which we have no reasonable explanation. We're attempting to answer questions like, "Why did this happen...?" *when we really don't know.*

    > IN THE OLD TESTAMENT, SICKNESS IS ALWAYS A CURSE AND HEALING IS ALWAYS A BLESSING.

  - Some pastors refer to these as "gap theories."[175] They are explanations we create to "fill in the gaps" between what the Bible says ("Jesus is our Healer") and our current experience ("Not everyone is healed."). We more readily create explanations- even bad ones- rather than living with the tension and simply saying, "I don't know why things are like this..."

---

[172] Hebrews 8:6, "But the ministry Jesus has received is as superior to theirs as the covenant of which he is mediator is superior to the old one, and it is founded on better promises" (NIV).

[173] 2 Corinthians 10:5 tells us to take every thought captive to the obedience of Christ. We do this by remembering that He has already completed our obedience- and done it thoroughly well.

[174] Many people believe that God is the One who causes chaos, inflicts people with disease, and sets up many of the trials we face in life. We do not see anything in the Bible to back this point-of-view. Rather, we see Jesus ministering total salvation to people in those situations.

[175] See "Closing the Gap on Healing," a message preached by Greg Haswell of Northlands Church in Atlanta, Georgia. Preached on 10-21-2012. The church's website is http://northlandschurch.com

- **Even the Bible has examples of people trying to explain calamity for which they have no explanation.** The Book of Job shows us how people did this thousands of years ago. Job suffered horrifically. He lost his family, his possessions, and his health. His friends urged him to confess his sin, that surely he had done something to cause this.[176]

  - Job continually argued that he had not- that he was righteous. He actually begged to take his case before God (see Job 31:35-37, for instance). He was certain that there was a mistake in the justice system somewhere, that he was getting what someone else deserved.

  - In all of this, one of Job's friends said the following: "Job uselessly opens his mouth and *multiplies words without knowledge* [drawing the worthless conclusion that the righteous have no more advantage than the wicked]" (Job 35:16 AMP, emphasis added).

  - His friends were certain he had sinned; he was certain that he hadn't.

  - Finally, God shows up and speaks to all of them, telling each of them that they are wrong. Amidst a lengthy speech, God Himself said this of Job, *to Job*: "Who is this that *darkens counsel by words without knowledge*" (38:2 AMP, emphasis added). That is, "You're speaking a lot and just confusing the issue... really you don't know what you're talking about!" Sometimes we do this with healing!

- **Remember that Jesus always sent His disciples out with the commission to heal- and the power to actually do it.** The assumption is that *people would be blessed.*

---

[176] Remarkably, Job happened in a time period in which Satan actually went into the presence of God (Job 1:6, 2:1). We know that this no longer happens, as Satan has been cast out of the presence of God (Isaiah 14:12f., Ezekiel 28:14f., Luke 10:18, Revelation 12:1f.). In other words, we shouldn't build our theology of healing and sickness on that book- which is what many Christians inadvertently do. The Cross changes everything.

- He sent the twelve out in Luke 9:1-2: "Then Jesus called together the Twelve [apostles] and gave them power and authority over all demons, and to **cure diseases**, 2 And He sent them out to announce and preach the kingdom of God and to **bring healing**" (AMP, emphasis added).

- He sent the seventy out in Luke 10:1-12. Notice what He says to them in Luke 10:8-9:"Whenever you go into a town and they receive and accept and welcome you, eat what is set before you; 9 And **heal the sick** in

> JESUS DIDN'T INSTRUCT HIS DISCIPLES ON HOW TO EXPLAIN THE CAUSES OF THE DIS-EASE; HE EMPOWERED THEM TO HEAL!

  it and say to them, The kingdom of God has come close to you" (AMP, emphasis mine).

- He sent all believers out in Mark 16:15-20. Remember what verse 18 says: "...they will lay their hands on the sick, and **they will get well**" (AMP, emphasis added).

- **In other words, Jesus didn't instruct His disciples on how to explain the causes of the dis-ease; He empowered them to heal!**[177]

5. Do not simply condemn the "_bad_ _fruit_." Seek to plant a _healthy_ _root_.

- **The fruit reveals the root.** The thing you "see" outside reveals something about the inside.

  - Diseased fruit- *whether it manifests as sickness, financial lack, relational strife, lack of purpose and direction, emotional*

---

[177] See earlier in the book regarding *therapeuo* and the mission of the disciples.

volatility, or any other bad fruit- is simply a result of the root which is feeding it.[178]

- Healthy fruit, on the other hand, is a result of the roots which are nourishing and giving life to it.

- **Dealing with fruit is *temporary-* addressing roots is *permanent.***

  - You can remove bad fruit from a "sick" person in the same way you can remove a bad apple from a diseased tree. But, that same fruit will return unless the roots change.

> THAT SAME FRUIT WILL RETURN UNLESS THE ROOTS CHANGE.

  - This is the reason so many people go "in and out" of rehabs. And it's the same reason many people return to destructive habits. Habits are simply *fruits*.[179]

  - On another level, this is the same reason people lose and gain weight repeatedly- or get out of debt, go back in, get out, go back in... The fruit is addressed without dealing with the root causes!

- **As well, there are an infinite number of fruits, but only a few roots. Keeping a list of all possible fruits is impossible; understanding the basic underlying roots is doable.[180]** This is especially true when you consider that the same fruit on two different people may have two *different* root causes.

---

[178] Stephen DeSilva's book *Money and the Prosperous Soul* is a great read on the roots of poverty.

[179] This is why we have spent so much time dealing with deeper theological issues (which are roots) during this study. To truly minister healing (a fruit), you need solid roots. Healing is a fruit of practicing *therapeuo*.

[180] I've got a theory I'm working through about all the side effects of pharmaceuticals. I think, many times, pharmaceuticals are only hitting symptoms in the body. When that one is covered up, a different symptom pops up to alert you to the fact that you've got a deeper issue going on. Think about it. Why else would there be so many possible side effects to a single issue? Because everyone's body is different, and everyone has different thoughts, emotions, and spiritual issues with which they're dealing. Oh... and that's just the physical issues related to the drugs. This doesn't include the emotional, financial, and relational roots.

- For example, one person may manifest envy (a work of the flesh, per Galatians 5:21) as a fruit of feeling unloved (isolated, abandonment). Another may manifest the same envy as a result of bitterness towards someone.

- Another example with the root of isolation / abandonment: one person may manifest this as an over-achiever, seeking to always been admired and desired by others. Another may manifest this as rebellion.

- **Many times, the fruit is simply a side effect or symptom of the real issue.** Can you heal a side effect? Or are you better off just going for the real, deeper matter?[181]

- **How do you know which root to go for?** *You listen...*

  - Many times the person will tell you how they feel... in doing so, they will reveal part of their story, highlighting things that need to be addressed. Remember, though, you are looking for roots- not fruits- as they do this.

  - Other times, the Lord will show you...

  - In either case, *listening* is an important skill (most ministers simply talk too much!).

- **A helpful hint? Always begin from the "inside out," addressing the value and worth of the person as a son or daughter of their Heavenly Father, who deeply adores them.**

  - Many times, physical symptoms will disappear when the deeper spiritual issues of identity are addressed.

  - Remember, harmful emotional experiences can be stored by the limbic system somewhere throughout the body. As the emotional wounds of the soul are healed, physical healing often follows. Forgiveness often brings instant healing.

---

[181] Henry Wright calls this "shadow boxing" with side effects (p95, *A More Excellent Way*).

Dis-eased Root = Dis-eased Fruit

LOOK BENEATH THE SURFACE TO ADDRESS THE REAL ISSUES

"It is obvious… repetitive, loveless, cheap sex; a stinking accumulation of mental and emotional garbage; frenzied and joyless grabs for happiness; trinket gods; magic-show religion; paranoid loneliness; cutthroat competition; all-consuming-yet-never-satisfied wants; a brutal temper; an impotence to love or be loved; divided homes and divided lives; small-minded and lopsided pursuits; the vicious habit of depersonalizing everyone into a rival; uncontrolled and uncontrollable addictions; ugly parodies of community. I could go on" (Galatians 5:19-21 MSG).

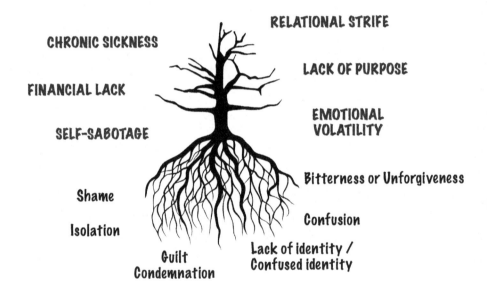

RELATIONAL STRIFE

CHRONIC SICKNESS

LACK OF PURPOSE

FINANCIAL LACK

EMOTIONAL VOLATILITY

SELF-SABOTAGE

Bitterness or Unforgiveness

Shame

Confusion

Isolation

Lack of identity / Confused identity

Guilt Condemnation

Note: the fruit we see is really a manifestation of the root issues. You will "see" many fruits. However, there are only a few major roots that you will face. If you can address these roots, the fruit will change.

Healthy Root = Healthy Fruit

CHANGE THE ROOTS AND THE FRUIT TRANSFORMS!

"He brings gifts into our lives, much the same way that fruit appears in an orchard—things like affection for others, exuberance about life, serenity. We develop a willingness to stick with things, a sense of compassion in the heart, and a conviction that a basic holiness permeates things and people. We find ourselves involved in loyal commitments, not needing to force our way in life, able to marshal and direct our energies wisely" (Galatians 5:22-23 MSG).

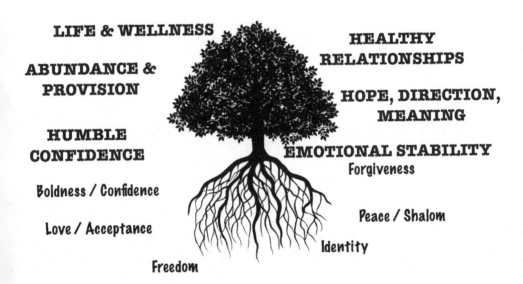

LIFE & WELLNESS

ABUNDANCE & PROVISION

HUMBLE CONFIDENCE

Boldness / Confidence

Love / Acceptance

Freedom

HEALTHY RELATIONSHIPS

HOPE, DIRECTION, MEANING

EMOTIONAL STABILITY
Forgiveness

Peace / Shalom

Identity

Note: On the illustration above, you'll see the healthy alternatives of the "bad fruits" on the opposite page. Remember, these are the result of the new roots, though- excellent fruit does not simply grow- or remain- on its own.

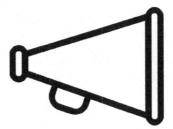

Apply Habit 3 & Tell

TOUCH THE BODY, SOUL, AND SPIRIT
YOU CARRY THE PRESENCE & POWER
FOCUS ON WHAT'S RIGHT

☐ We spent much time dealing with core theological issues (roots) in the beginning of this study. Ministering healing to others, I believe, is a fruit. Walking in healing- *therapeuo*- is also a fruit. Do you agree or disagree? And why...?

FRUIT:
Walking in healing, ministering healing

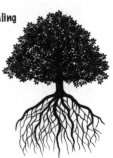

ROOT:
What I believe about God, faith, and healing

☐ Two roots we've discussed throughout the book are identity and forgiveness. Describe the importance of each- and how they effect all of life (i.e., look at the bad root of lack of identity / confused identity and bitterness / unforgiveness; compare them to identity and peace / shalom).

☐ Proverbs tells us that "A sound heart is the life of the flesh; but envy the rottenness of the bones" (Proverbs 14:30 KJV). We discussed how the bone marrow supports the cardiovascular system and the immune system, where we discussed the emotions and frequencies). So, we see a glimpse of scientific truth here in the Bible. As well, as read that laughter actually strengthens the immune system (see Proverbs 17:22). What does this communicate to you about the "joy of the Lord" being your strength (Nehemiah 8:10)? Is this just an emotional idea, or is it really a physical reality that has everything to do with *therapeuo*?

☐ In this chapter we discussed that "you are a source" of the Kingdom's presence and power. To come in contact with Heaven, people simply need to encounter you. In what way does this effect your theology? And how many times have you lived from a "cistern" theology (one that says "I've got to go get refilled- I'm empty!) or a "well" theology ("Oh, no! I'm not connected to a source!"). If you are a "fountain" or "spring," you never run dry. What do you think?

☐ I mentioned three causes of illness- sin, Satan, and "something else." How does this fit with the chart we created earlier in the book about toxins and deficiencies? Where does *therapeuo* fit into the three? How do you reconcile the two charts below?

Two Causes of Disease...Naturally

	TOXICITY	DEFICIENCY
THIS MEANS	My body comes in contact with things that it does not need, things which are harmful to it	My body is not receiving some of the things it does need, things which would benefit it
EXAMPLES INCLUDE	Sugar, artificial sweeteners, cigarette smoke, high fructose corn syrup, gluten, etc. (note: stress is a factor here, too!)	Dehydration, lack of sleep / rest, calcium deficiency, exercise / movement
SOLUTION INCLUDES	Purity- eliminating toxins whenever possible	Supplement- flooding my body with nutrients and other things that boost my wellness

Causes of Dis-ease... Spiritually

IF YOU SUGGEST...	THEY MAY FEEL...
SIN	Condemned
SATAN	Alarmed
SOMETHING ELSE	Confused
GOD	Unloved

☐ How do you resist created "gap theories" when you don't have a reason for why you- or someone else- isn't healed? And why do we have the tendency to put everything into tidy theological and philosophical boxes? Are you really OK with some ambiguity?

APPLY HABIT 3 & TELL

☐ Remember, when you are ministering to someone, you don't have to communicate everything the Lord gives you in that moment.[182] Many times He'll impart information for you to help you better love them. Why is it important to be able to discern what's for you and what's for them? How can you grow in this area?

☐ Reaping and sowing is a concept that factors into *therapeuo*. Often, the results of lifestyle choices don't manifest quickly. Sometimes, they do. I was 50 pounds overweight- and got that way by gaining 3 pounds / year for just over 16 years. That breaks down to *only* about 1/4 pound per month. It was so slow I never noticed it until my body had changed dramatically- and my health had deteriorated. At the same time, when I began losing the weight, it was gradual (thankfully, a lot faster to lose it than to gain it!). I didn't notice the day-to-day change at all. My wife, however, noticed after one week. Why, then, is persistence important when we take action? In what ways does this encourage you? Does it frustrate you?

---

[182] Graham Cooke's book *Approaching the Heart of Prophecy* is an incredible resource that discusses this topic in more detail.

APPLY HABIT 3 & TELL

☐ What does it mean that *"You don't need the cause; you just need the cure!"*?
Three things can cause the need for healing: sin, Satan, or something else.
Really, in this question, we're talking about your stance when something falls in
the third category- *"something else"*- and you don't know how to reconcile it.

☐ Why do we tend to attribute things to God (like illness) instead of crediting
them to the Devil? And why do we credit things to the Devil (i.e., prosperity,
abundance) that are likely gifts and blessings from God- according to
Deuteronomy 28? Why do we get our theological lines crossed on some major
issues? And, in what ways does this effect us on a deeper level?

☐ I love this quote: "God's perfect will is not to heal you; His perfect will is that
you don't get sick" (Henry Wright). Here's how I interpret it:

- Get well now (*iaomai* or *therapeuo*)

- Avoid future sickness by sowing wellness now (*therapeuo*)

I'd love to know your thoughts...

APPLY HABIT 3 & TELL

☐ Throughout this book we've talked about identity. Sometimes, we get our identity confused. In fact, I believe a lack of identity / confused identity is one of the destructive roots that manifests itself as unhealthy fruits. What part of the Cross wasn't enough for you and your transformed identity? What part wasn't enough for the people you will serve?

☐ We discussed seven things that raise your frequency higher above the wellness line. What stood out the most to you? What seemed surprising? What are your next steps to leverage what you've learned?

☐ Is it a sin to not choose *therapeuo*? By now, you know that my heart is unbalanced grace- so there's no condemnation coming from me on this issue. I'm simply looking for your opinion.

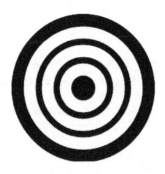

6. Review the 3 Habits

DEAL WITH YOU
REVIEW WHAT YOU'VE LEARNED
GET THE TOOLS YOU NEED SUCCEED

"Choose life..." (Deuteronomy 30:19).

"Now may the God of peace Himself sanctify your completely... your whole spirit, soul, and body..." (1 Thessalonians 5:23 NKJV).

"He who raised Christ from the dead will also give life to your mortal bodies through His spirit who dwells in you" (Romans 8:11 NKJV).

A. Deal with __you__.

- The greatest work your Father will do in your world is the work He's going to do, first of all, directly to you.

- Everything else is simply an overflow- and is secondary- to that.

1. God generally does something __to____you__before doing something __through__ __you__.

- **Paul is clear that we don't serve God in other way other relationships are served.** He says, "Human hands can't serve his needs--for He has no needs. He himself gives life and breath to everything, and He satisfies every need" (Acts 17:25 NLT).

- **Think about it this way: Jesus said, "You cannot serve God and Mammon" (Matthew 6:24).**

  - When people serve money, they don't try to meet money's needs. Rather, they position themselves to benefit from money- *to receive!*

    > AS WE RECEIVE, WE ARE ABLE TO BECOME CONDUITS- AND TO PASS THAT GOODNESS TO OTHERS.

  - In the same manner, the way to serve God best is to position yourself to *receive* from Him- not to give.

- **As we *receive*, we become conduits- and we pass that goodness to others.**

NEXT STEPS

2. Your ___underlying___ ___beliefs___ will effect your posture.

- **Communication experts suggest 90% of all communication is non-verbal!** In other words, the old adage is true: It's not *what* you say, it's *how* you say it.

- If you carry unresolved feelings about the goodness of God, if you don't have the "faith issue" in check, and if you doubt His desire to heal... this will "come out" in how you communicate with people- even if you say the right things. **Make sure you have a foundation on all the "think right" issues we discussed- about God, about faith, and about healing!**

3. Walk in ___health___ / ___therapeuo___ as your own lifestyle choice.

- **First, this will give you more confidence, affecting your posture.**

- **Second, as most communication is non-verbal, it will give credibility to your message.** In a real sense, the message and the messenger are inseparable.

- **Third, your ministry will be limited by your physical body.** It is the "container" for your soul and spirit. You cannot do all of the incredible things the Lord has in store for you if you are sick and tired on the couch.

4. Remember that your Father generally expresses Himself ___through___ ___people___.

- **The Holy Spirit is more passionate to touch people with the Father's heart that you are.**

> AS WE RECEIVE, WE ARE ABLE TO BECOME CONDUITS- AND TO PASS THAT GOODNESS TO OTHERS.

  - "Can you bat the Holy Spirit into the upper deck of a baseball stadium?"

    - I asked this question to Kent Mattox, pastor of Word Alive Church in Coldwater, Alabama. Before starting his own church, he traveled with Benny Hinn (a healing evangelist). I'd heard rumors of Benny actually "batting the Holy Spirit" during a crusade. Apparently, Benny stood onstage near the pitcher's mound (the story goes). There were people in the "cheap seats" needing a touch of God, so he pretended to loft a baseball in the air- just like you do when you're pitching it up to yourself to then swing and pop it with the bat. Then, he actually took a pretend swing. Remarkably, second laters, people in the upper deck fell over as if they were touched by the Spirit.

    - Whether this actually happened or not, I don't know. But, I wanted to know if it was possible. Kent said he never saw *that* happen, but that he saw many things that were... well... *interesting...*

  - "Here's what I've learned," he said. "The Holy Spirit desperately wants to touch people- and to give them an expression of the Father's love. So, He'll back you up and do just about anything you want to do..."

- **This story was a game-changer for me.** God is simply looking for people to express Himself through! He will back me up when I step out in faith!

- If my ability to reach people is dependent upon me & my gifts, sometimes it will work and other times it won't.

- However, if my ability is dependent on God's heart to simply love His children... and if the expression of that love doesn't require a formula but just a venue to express Himself (in a way that I can actually choose), then I know He will "show up" every single time.

> IF MY ABILITY IS DEPENDENT ON GOD'S HEART TO SIMPLY LOVE HIS CHILDREN... I KNOW HE WILL "SHOW UP" EVERY SINGLE TIME.

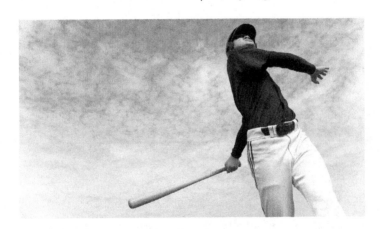

B. ___Review___ what you have ___learned___ - the 3 habits.

- **Habits are actions that happen naturally- almost without thinking about them.** No one reminds us to look in the rearview mirror before putting our car into reverse. No one reminds us to tie our shoes after we put them on. Or to brush our teeth before bed. These things happen naturally, as an overflow of our regular routine. In fact, something feels "off" when we accidentally forget any of these small, mundane activities.

- **My prayer is that the 3 habits will occur naturally for us, too...**

  - That we will *think* the right things about our Father, about faith, and about healing...

  - That we will *touch* others... embracing the goodness of our Father and everything He has provided to us for health and wellness... and expressing that to others...

  - That we will express that with confidence... and *tell* others of His goodness, calling forth the greatness within each of them.

Review of the 3 Habits

HABIT		ACTION
👑	THINK	Belief / foundation
🔲	TOUCH	Connection / intimacy
📢	TELL	Prayer / expression

- **If you identify a "hole" in your approach to others, then you can use the grid on the following page to find out how to resolve it.**

- *If you feel that there's no foundation to what you're doing*, go back and work on the "think" habit. Review the notes about God's goodness, about faith, and about Biblical healing.

- *If you feel there's a disconnect between you and the people to whom you're ministering* (such that the exchange seems more like you're just relaying raw information rather than genuinely connecting with people- it lacks intimacy, in other words), review the notes on touch. Remember, most conversation is non-verbal. *Touch* communicates. Maybe you need to anoint them with more fervor and confidence. Perhaps you need to learn more about a few of the oils. Also, you can "warm up" the person by shaking hands, hugging, and touching them before the ministry exchange formally begins.

- *If you sense that you're hitting a wall, that chains aren't being broken…* perhaps you lack expression. If this happens, review the *tell* information. Remember to declare truth to the whole person- body, soul, and spirit. Focus on planting good roots which will result in good fruits- and a bountiful harvest.

All 3 Are Important

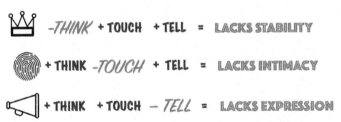

-THINK + TOUCH + TELL = LACKS STABILITY

+ THINK *-TOUCH* + TELL = LACKS INTIMACY

+ THINK + TOUCH − *TELL* = LACKS EXPRESSION

Note What are you missing? See where you need to focus. Then begin "working on yourself" (as we discussed in A. of this chapter) first. The results will come. Compare with the graphics earlier in the book, as well.

C. Get the __tools__ you need to be __successful__.

- **Teaching materials.** There are a few versions of this material available for you.

  - *Live workshop.* You can study with others in a familiar setting and then actually practice.

  - *Online course.* You can study on your own, or even watch the videos with a group of friends. As well, you can use the online material to review what you learned in person.

- **Your oils.** In the appendix of this book, I'll provide you with instructions on how to order your own *now*.[183]

---

[183] See the appendix chapter, "Start Your Own."

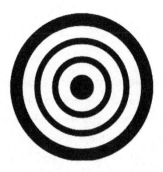

Apply the 3 Habits

DEAL WITH YOU
REVIEW WHAT YOU'VE LEARNED
GET THE TOOLS YOU NEED TO SUCCEED

☐ A few times in this book we've talked about the greatest work the Lord does in your world being the work that He does *in* you. What do you make of this?

☐ What are some of your underlying beliefs that have changed as a result of this study? This may include how you view Father God, how you view faith, or how you see healing- as well as other areas that may have changed for you. In what ways is this a good thing for you? What has stretched you the most?

☐ I shared my conversation with pastor Kent Mattox during this chapter- where Kent told me that God is desperately looking for people to express His love through. To me, this means that if you want to heal, you can heal. If you want to pray and bless, you can pray and bless. If you want to share prophesy, you can... In what ways does this concept give you more confidence as a son or daughter?

☐ We discussed that you can see the "weak point" in your ministry and easily determine the area you need to focus. For instance, if you lack foundation and stability, look at your belief system (*think*). If you're not connecting with others, evaluate your confidence with *touch* (i.e., laying on of hands, anointing, the oils). And, if you lack expression and feel you aren't communicating, review *tell* (See the graphic below).

Where are you the strongest? The weakest? Where do you have the most experience? The least?

All 3 Are Important

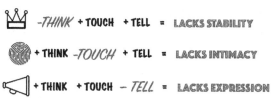

-*THINK* + TOUCH + TELL = LACKS STABILITY

+ THINK -*TOUCH* + TELL = LACKS INTIMACY

+ THINK + TOUCH − *TELL* = LACKS EXPRESSION

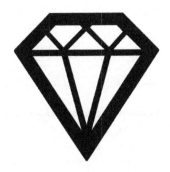

7. Step-by-Step Healing Model

AN ENVIRONMENT OF EASE & EXPECTATION

LEVELS OF ANOINTING

STEP-BY-STEP

"Do not neglect the spiritual gift within you..." (1 Timothy 4:14).

A. Creating an environment of expectation and ease involves your personal __beliefs__ & __behaviors__.

- Let's look at our beliefs and behaviors, first. Then, we'll discuss how everyone can do this!

- Finally, we'll walk through the step-by-step healing model.

1. God generally does something _to_ _you_ before doing something _through you_ (beliefs).

- **The more of His heart you catch, the more you'll be able to communicate with others.**[184]

    - Again, most communication is non-verbal.

    - One thing I'm learning here is that, yes, better communicators (and more gifted communicators) usually have "better words." But, since up to 90% of the communication process is non-verbal, it's the non-verbal that sets the environment. It's the non-verbal that raises the level of receptivity of the hearers.

    > THE MORE OF HIS HEART YOU CATCH, THE MORE YOU'LL BE ABLE TO COMMUNICATE WITH OTHERS.

- **When the Father gives us a true heart for people, they tangibly feel that.** *Love communicates.* Whatever He does to us, is going to shine through us.

2. As well, you'll develop more _skill_ and _confidence_ in this area the more you _do_ _it_ (behaviors).

- Oddly enough, a lot of people *think* you either "have it" or "you don't," that is, you can either pray for healing (and see people healed) or you can't. **However, anyone can pray for healing. The commission and power were given to *all* of Jesus' disciples!**

---

[184] Yes, we've hit the concept a few times in the material- but it's foundational!

- I still pray for people and they're not healed. Then I pray for others and they are. The same will be true for you, too, and **you'll see your success rate elevate with time and practice.**[185]

- If it doesn't work, it doesn't mean you don't have the ability to heal:

  - We have 9 kids. Two are adopted (they joined our family when they were 7 & 5). We've taught 7 of the children how to walk. Every single one of them- *without exception*- fell the first few times they tried. In fact, they fell more than they actually walked. Yet, at no time did we ever think, "Oh, this one must not have the ability to walk…"

  - No, because we know the norm is that people do walk. Non-walkers are the exception.

  - I believe the same is true of healing. It is an empowerment given my Jesus in the Great Commission (see Mark 16:15f.). He actually commanded His disciples to do this every time He sent them out. It's just something that may take practice.

> YOU'LL SEE YOUR SUCCESS RATE GO UP WITH TIME AND PRACTICE.

- **This is true with most spiritual things we do.** Even preachers learn to communicate better (ever heard your pastor's first sermon? It was probably… well… not as good as the ones you hear now!). Healing is the same. You may have to crawl before you walk… and walk before you run.

---

[185] Think about it this way: your pastor's first sermon was probably horrible! Yet with prayer and practice, everything has gotten much better! No doubt, your pastor is spiritually gifted in this area- and called. But, it took time and practice to develop the skills that God had given. Give yourself the same grace to grow!

- Honestly, though, I'm surprise at how quickly people acquire this skill.[186]

- That said, let's look at the next point, because there are some things we need to acknowledge about giftedness...

B. There are different levels of __anointing__ (read: God-given skill), but everyone can __heal__.

1. Some people just do it __better__.

- **One pastor suggests we should acknowledge there are different levels of gifting in the healing ministry.** This is wise. Some people are more gifted at teaching; others are more gifted in evangelism or acts of service. We don't get frustrated about it- we simply leverage those gifts, letting others participate, too.

---

[186] Now, inevitably someone brings up the issue about giftedness and skill. I tell them that, "Yes, God gifts people in different ways. We see that throughout the Bible. However, part of the Great Commission is for all disciples to pray for healing. Jesus said they would. So, we can assume that healing will come." When I've tried this in public venues where I'm teaching, it *always* comes, in fact.

- We've seen people healed of hepatitis, which was caught through drug use with needles.

- We've seen a man walk who had a tumor on his leg and had been unable to walk. Ironically, he had no faith at all and became "proof" to others that faith isn't a requirement.

- We've seen heartbeats that were irregular move into perfect sync.

- We've seen backs and shoulders and other sore parts healed.

Oddly enough, in many of these cases it was residents at rehabilitation / reentry ministry I used to lead who were praying for other residents as we coach them along. To me, this shows everyone that it's not contingent on being a staff leader at a ministry. Or even be far along in your walk. Or have had a perfect day. Or have even (get this) prayed that day! Healing is given to everyone. Anyone can be healed; everyone can pray.

- Jack Deere says, "We can admit to varying degrees of intensity and quality in gifts of evangelism, in gifts of teaching, and in other gifts. Why can't we do that with the gift of healing? Or the gift of miracles? Or the gift of prophecy?"[187] As such, **we will expect some people to have a "greater frequency" of healing. Yet we can all do it- and should.**

- Now, some of the categories in the chart which follows are undeniably abused. However, that doesn't make them less true. In fact, you might actually argue that it makes the "truth of them" more true. **You can't counterfeit something that doesn't exist.** You can only counterfeit an authentic, original.

> "WE CAN ADMIT TO VARYING DEGREES OF INTENSITY AND QUALITY... IN OTHER GIFTS. WHY CAN'T WE DO THAT WITH THE GIFT OF HEALING?"

- As well, though people are sometimes skeptical about Divine Healing, **it's important to realize that everyone is usually open to being prayed for- regardless of their theology. "**

    - Everyone really believes in the importance of healing. We have hospitals and a medical profession because people believe in the importance of healing."[188]

    - When they- or a loved one (particularly a family member)- is sick, their theology always becomes a bit more open.

---

[187] Jack Deere, *Surprised by the Holy Spirit*, p67.

[188] Jack Deere, *Surprised by the Power of the Holy Spirit*, Kindle location 2420.

Various Levels of Anointing for Healing

VARIOUS LEVELS	DESCRIBED	BIBLICAL EXAMPLE
IN YOU	Jesus said that all believers can lay hands on the sick and they will recover. This power is given to all followers of Jesus because the Spirit is in them / they all have the life of Christ.	Mark 16:15-20. Jesus commissioned all disciples, saying that people will be healed by each of them.
ON YOU	When the anointing is "on you" it transfers from you to other things that touch you.	Acts 19:11f. says that unusual miracles were performed by Paul. Handkerchiefs and aprons that touched him would be taken to the sick, laid on them, and they would recover. The anointing jumped from him to it to them, traveling like static electricity.
AROUND YOU	When the anointing is "around you" it changes the atmosphere. The entire environment is different, such that people are healed just by coming near.	Acts 5:15 tells us that when Peter walked by people that were under his shadow would be healed. As such, people began carrying the sick and setting them in places where they knew he would be.

2. Even if they're not __healed__, don't stop praying for __healing__.

- **The reality is that everyone isn't healed.** Jesus sometimes waits until heaven to heal people. We need to acknowledge that. Again, it is this tension that causes us to often create the "gap theories."

- **Because some people are not healed, some opponents of healing suggest that healing must not be God's will.** Think about from another angle that you already understand and embrace.

  > EVERYONE IS USUALLY OPEN TO BEING PRAYED FOR- REGARDLESS OF THEIR THEOLOGY.

  - The Bible tells us that it *is* His will that *all* people be saved. 1 Timothy 2:3-4 says to pray for the salvation of all men precisely because it is His will: "For such [praying] is good and right, and [it is] pleasing and acceptable to God our Savior, 4 Who wishes all men to be saved and [increasingly] to perceive and recognize and discern and know precisely and correctly the [divine] Truth" (AMP). Notice, it is His will- *and* He asks us to pray for their salvation even though not all people get saved.

  - He states that this is clearly His will in another passage as well: 2 Peter 3:9 tells us that He is not willing that *any* should perish but that all should come to eternal life.

  - Even so, people still reject Jesus' grace and salvation.

- **We can argue the same about healing- some receive, others don't. It doesn't negate the Father's heart, though.**[189]

  - We pray total healing. Just as Jesus died on the Cross for the forgiveness of the sins of all people, Jesus bled for the healing of all people (Psalm 103:3).

---

[189] And, remember, we don't have to create a theological box to explain something that we don't yet understand.

- Not everyone is healed; not everyone is saved. But we still contend for both![190]

We Still Pray for Both

REALITY	BUT WE WILL PRAY FOR...	GOD'S DESIRE?
EVERYONE IS NOT SAVED	We still pray for everyone, and tell people about Jesus... we don't know who will be saved.	God desires for all to be saved (1 Timothy 2:3-4, 2 Peter 3:9).
EVERYONE IS NOT HEALED	We still pray, knowing that the Kingdom touches and heals some.	Does God desire healing for us in the same? I believe He does...

C. Just walk it out- general instructions for praying __healing__ / __wholeness__ for someone.

1. Realize where you __stand__.

- **You have authority to heal** (Mark 16:15-20. See also Mark 3:14f., Matthew 10:1f.). And, you are praying from the third realm, from Heaven, where there is perfect healing.

- **You are praying *from* victory- not praying *for* victory.** Jesus is seated in Heaven- and your spirit is, right now, seated with Him (see Ephesians 1:20, Ephesians 2:6).

- **A few important activities are already happening- you simply join them when you pray for healing!**

---

[190] We discussed this concept of intimacy and health earlier in the book.

- Jesus is interceding for you and the person to whom you are ministering (Hebrews 7:25, Romans 8:34).

  - The Holy Spirit intercedes at the same time (Romans 8:26), specifically that all things will work together for the good (Romans 8:28).

> YOUR PRAYER IS NOT THE FIRST THING TO HAPPEN ON BEHALF OF YOU OR THE PERSON TO WHOM YOU ARE MINISTERING...

  - When you pray, you jump into this huddle, in partnership with what is already happening.

- **It is Jesus' predisposition to minister healing- not to withhold it** (3 John 2). We have made this clear in this chapter (and in the chapter about *Think*).

2. Remove the __barriers__ to belief.

- **The barrier may be a physical situation, the environment, etc.**

  - Jesus sent the mourners out of the home when praying for Jairus' dead daughter (Mark 5:40).

  - Peter later did the same thing when a woman in the early church died (Acts 9:40). Note, too, that when he prayed (read the passage carefully), he could not even look at her as he prayed. After praying, he turned *towards* her and told her to rise. Her dead body was a barrier- so he looked in the opposite direction to pray.

  - Elijah prayed for a drought to come. Three years later he prayed for it to rain. While praying, he buried his head between his knees as he bowed to the ground. And, he sent someone else to investigate the environment, to see if rain was coming. He sent them seven times while he built his faith and prayed without looking (1 Kings 18:42-43).

- If something is hindering your ability to pray (whether it is the environment, a sound you hear, something you see, whatever), simply make the adjustments you need to make and push through.

YOU JOIN SOMETHING ALREADY HAPPENING

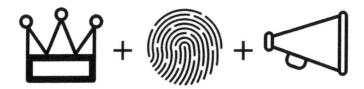

JESUS	HOLY SPIRIT	YOU
Hebrews 7:25	Romans 8:26-28	Mark 16:18
Romans 8:34		

Note: your prayer is not the first thing to happen on behalf of you or the person to whom you are ministering. Jesus has already died for them, purchasing their sozo. And, He and the Holy Spirit pray even now. You join this... from the place of victory!

All 3 Are Important

 JESUS = THE TRUTH, THE REVELATION WE THINK UPON...

 HOLY SPIRIT = THE TOUCH, THE EXPRESSION OF GOD

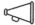 YOU = THE ONE WHO TELLS- DECLARES- THE FATHER'S HEART

3. The person to whom you are ministering may carrying the ___barrier___.

- **People carry a lot of theological barriers with them.** They believe the wrong things about God (i.e., that He caused their sickness), they believe the wrong things about faith (i.e., the reason they are sick is because they don't have enough), or they believe the wrong things about healing (they've disconnected the miraculous from "walking out" healing every single day).[191] Or, they may not yet be ready to get rid of the old, sick identity- as odd as this sounds.

> ... THEY SENSE THE LORD'S UNCONDITIONAL LOVE AND GRACE, MANY TIMES HEALING WILL COME INSTANTLY...

  - Most often, they believe these the first two because they've been taught bad theology about God and faith by well-meaning church leaders.

  - Oddly enough, health (the third issue) is rarely discussed in the church.[192]

  - As well, it seems we've moved from talking about our true identity to more "practical" topics.

---

[191] If you pray healing for someone with diabetes but they persist in eating junk, they may believe that healing doesn't happen when, really, they negated the healing by choosing not to make adjustments in their lifestyle. Remember, *therapeuo* is almost always accompanied by action. The same is true with obese people- and the myriad of associated health issues that arise... like I personally experienced... Many times people will give you excuses as to why the can't exercise, why they must continued eating diet foods (which are unhealthy, highly processed, and can't be digested by the body). These are instances of mental disconnects in our belief system about the full scope of healing. Remember, if you win the lottery and don't know how to manage money, statistics say you'll be broke in 18 months. If you receive Divine healing (*iaomai*), but don't accompany it with lifestyle choices (*therapeuo*), the healing may prove inconsequential.

[192] Seriously, when is the last time you heard a sermon, Bible study, or small group discussed related to health? Why do we give this aspect of our lives away to big Pharma, the health club, etc.?

- **Do not condemn them** (by blaming the situation on their sin), **do not make them afraid** (by blaming it on Satan), **do not make them feel unloved** (by suggesting it is God who is causing them to be sick).

  - **If you address any of the above, do so gently.**

  - **People already feel condemned, afraid, and unloved.** If you can shepherd them through the Gospel, such that they sense the Lord's unconditional love and grace, many times healing will come *instantly* without much prayer. Remember, harmful emotional wounds are stored by the limbic system throughout the body. Healing an emotional or spiritual wound may actually alleviate the manifesting illness (which is, in this case, simply a symptom of something deeper).

  - **Many times, I've seen that "making light" of the situation disarms everything and raises everyone's faith.**

    - I may mention that I'm not going to take the credit if something great happens- and I know they won't- so, on the flip-side, we both agree that we won't take any blame for anything that doesn't happen, either.

    - This helps, because many times people feel they've done something wrong which has caused their condition. And, they sense that they're responsible. Removing this burden quickly eliminates the obstacles to healing.

4. Find Scripture that "builds your case" and "supports your request" to the Lord.

- **Scripture builds faith.** Testimonies you know of other people who've experienced the same thing they see in the Bible builds faith. Here, we're not using the Bible to "prove" to God that He's obligated to do something. He's already shown us His desire to bless His people. We're using the Scripture to *change us*, to encourage ourselves![193]

- That said, **note in the Bible where there are similar situations to what you are praying and asking the Lord to do- and stand on those Scriptures.** Build your faith- and theirs. Faith is not a work, but it can change the environment radically![194]

- As well, "Don't ever try to talk God into healing someone because that sick person deserves it. No one is healed because they deserve it. We are healed only because of the goodness of the Son of God."[195] Now, this may sound odd- but, remember, **if healing is based on what we deserve, their faith may erode depending on their emotional state at that moment.** They may feel like they don't deserve to be healed. Then, self-doubt, condemnation, and the accusations of the enemy can enter.

5. (You may need to then) __call__ __it__ into existence / " __claim__ __it__ " / __command__ ____it__ to happen!

- **There are many examples of people boldly proclaiming a new reality throughout Scripture:**[196]

    - Ezekiel and the dry bones (Ezekiel 37:1f.). Ezekiel stands in the valley of dry bones. The Lord asks him if the bones can

---

[193] Many times, a testimony will carry the same anointing as the original event it points to. Stories are that powerful. People see in others what's possible for them (Revelation 12:11).

[194] Earlier we discussed seven things that raise your frequency and push you above the wellness line. One is thoughts, another is emotions. Which one of these is faith? Is it a thought? A feeling? Either way, it sets things in motion…

[195] See Jack Deere's book, *Surprised by the Power of the Holy Spirit*, Kindle location 2506.

[196] Prophecy helps with healing; healing assists with prophecy. The concept of "teaching for life" helps with prophecy, etc. See The Kingdom 101 in the supplemental bonus material of the online class for more.

live. Ezekiel does what we most often do, telling the Lord that "You alone know." God then flips it on him, telling him- "You command it to happen. Tell them to rise up and come to life."

- Elijah and the rain (1 Kings 17:1f., 1 Kings 18:41f.). He called for rain, even though the Bible does not mention God ever telling him to do this (the same is true for calling fire down on the altar with the prophets of Baal. James 5:17-18 emphasizes that Elijah was a human- just like us- inferring that we should do the same.

- Paul at Lystra with the crippled man (Acts 14:9- note, his message of identity, life and grace in Acts 13:39f.). He had to "speak" the healing once he "saw" it in his spirit.

- Peter and the beggar (Acts 3:5f.). Peter simply commanded the man to rise, then pulled him to his feet.

- Read the Gospels and count how many times Jesus prayed for healing as opposed to how many times He commanded it to happen by speaking it into existence![197]

- In other words, **your Father may actually want you to speak life into the situation.**[198] We could learn a great deal from the "name it and claim it" segment of the Church, in other words. Rather than belittling the misuses of the revelation they have received, we should learn the truth of what they have been given- and then use it![199]

  - "Sound has always been and continues to be one of the most important forces God ever created."[200]

---

[197] I don't know of any instances where He prayed and didn't command the healing to happen.

[198] Jesus said you won't have to ask Him for anything (John 16:23-24). He even taught the disciples to go straight to the Father (Matthew 6:9). This goes back to the core idea of understanding who God is.

[199] Remember the story about "batting the Holy Spirit"? Step out- God's got your back!

[200] Ray Hughes, p70 in chapter 7, "Sound of Heaven / Symphony of Earth" of The Physics of Heaven.

- Use the power of your sound to tell reality what to do!

6. Sometimes, an ___action___ is needed.

- Action is sometimes required by people who are being healed- especially when we're looking at the experience of *therapeuo-* of lifestyle healing. However, this might happen with *iaomai*, too. They are told to "take up their bed," to "rise and walk," or to do something specific. Though this is not always possible (i.e., someone being healed of cancer will not "rise and walk," they will go back to the doctor and have an MRI and further tests to confirm), it is good to note that **immediate action that is specific to the healing may actually reinforce what is being done.** This does not mean that they earn their healing anymore than we earn our forgiveness. However, the action does show they are walking in a new way- just as baptism shows you have identified with a new pattern of life.

> IMMEDIATE ACTION THAT IS SPECIFIC TO THE HEALING MAY ACTUALLY REINFORCE WHAT IS BEING DONE...

GOD GIVES A **DIRECTION**

PEOPLE WHO TAKE **ACTION**

EXPERIENCE A **MIRACLE**

- **Every time God gave someone a direction, those who took action experienced a miracle.** You see this theme of direction-action-miracle throughout the Bible:

  - The Children of Israel are told to walk into the Jordan River at flood stage, while carrying the Ark of the Covenant, before the waters subside. This would have been extremely dangerous- but it was the act of faith required of them (Joshua 3:8f.).

  - Namaan the Leper was healed after he agreed- *and acted-* on the command to wash himself in the Jordan River (see 2 Kings 5:1f., specifically 5:14). It is interesting that he at first dissented to this.

  - Jesus commanded the lepers to go show themselves to the priest after He healed all ten of them. The Bible is clear that they were healed "as they went" in obedience (Luke 17:14).

  > YOU SEE THIS THEME OF DIRECTION-ACTION-MIRACLE THROUGHOUT THE BIBLE...

  - Jesus commanded the paralytic to "rise and walk" (Mark 2:11-12).

  - Jesus told the blind man to wash the mud off his eyes- and then he could see (John 9:1f.).

  - Peter took the lame beggar by his hand, pulled him to his feet, and urged him to walk (Acts 3:6-7).

  - Aeneus, a man who had been paralyzed for eight years, was commanded by Peter to pick up his bed and walk (Acts 9:34-35).

  - Paul told the man in Lystra who had been crippled from birth to rise and walk (Acts 14:10).

- Earlier, **I told you my own story of walking in *therapeuo*- and how many health breakthroughs came instantly, while others came in their own time.** It's important that you don't ignore a direction that's been given to you! (Or one that's been given to you to give to them!)

THERAPEUO = ACTION
(BECAUSE IT IS A LIFESTYLE CHOICE)

7. A commonly asked question: Do you have to be ___present___ to minister healing to someone? Can somebody just "___stand___ ___in___" for someone else?

- **The answers are varied- even from the Bible:**

  - Jesus was *not* always present when He prayed for healing (i.e., the centurion's servant in Luke 7:1-10; the Syrophoenician woman's daughter in Mark 7:25-30).

  - Jesus *most often* was present, however (and even when He wasn't, He never had anyone "stand in." He just proclaimed healing).

  - Jesus was specific about being present, too. He addressed particular needs. Note, He actually *touched* lepers (who were forbidden to be touched, according to the Law), even though He regularly healed with just a word / command.

  - Since ministry is relational, it makes sense that the Lord would work through people to reach other people (so, touch them, hug them, love them physically, even).

- **Laying on of hands (and anointing) is helpful- though not a formula** (note: there is another lesson devoted only to a brief overview of the laying on of hands).[201]

- **If you have the ability to minister to someone in person, *do it*.** If not, pray for a "long distance" miracle- or even declare it- as we see Jesus regularly do![202]

- Notice how Jesus' brother emphasizes "in person" ministry: James 5:13-15 says, "Is anyone among you suffering? Let him pray. Is anyone cheerful? Let him sing psalms. **Is anyone among you sick? Let him call for the elders of the church, and let them pray over him, anointing him with oil in the name of the Lord.** And the prayer of faith will save the sick, and the Lord will raise him up. And if he has committed sins, he will be forgiven" (NKJV).

- **Also, think about the relational dynamic of healing:**

  - If sin has been the issue, it helps for people to feel accepted, etc. This removes another barrier to their healing (i.e., isolation). And, if you accept them, *they will feel accepted by God.*

  - Other notes on relational aspects: see Mark 3:14f., Matthew 10:1f. Notice that Jesus sent His disciples out. He presumably did this so they could be *present* to the people that they were going to reach- and touch. He could have instructed them to remain in a room and simply pray from afar if that was the model He wanted to emphasize.

- In the end, sometimes you just "go for it." **Your Heavenly Father is good and loves His children. The Kingdom is coming present- we**

---

[201] This chapter and a teaching video on the topic are both available in the bonus materials of the online version of this book.

[202] If you have the ability to pray for church members who are in the hospital by actually visiting them in person, then do it! Long term, I believe people are likely to be more readily healed by 1) laying on of hands and 2) training in *therapeuo* instead of 1) just visiting them in person and 2) praying from afar with a list.

get to bring it with us. And, you remember that "the anointing to heal and bring deliverance will be of no value in Heaven. These graces must be used here and now as part of the package of tools used to bring the nations to Jesus."[203]

8. By the way, ___**therapeuo**___ is your destiny. When you choose wellness, you enjoy the presence of the future ___**now**___!

- **Look back at the tree of life.**
  - The Old Testament says that all plants were given for *oklah*—for food and healing (see Genesis 1:29, Ezekiel 47:12).
  - The New Testament tells us that the leaves of the tree of life are for the *therapeuo* of the nations (Revelation 22:2).
- **Yes, we pray for miracles (*iaomai*). At the same time, we walk towards our destiny as we seek miraculous intervention.**

[203] Bill Johnson, *Release the Power of Jesus*, Kindle location 301.

Practical Overview of the 3 Habits

Before you begin, say your name (if you don't already know them... reach out and touch them, shaking their hand- or even hugging them, as appropriate). Note: just continually move through the same process that we learned in the book: Think, Touch, Tell. If you can remember these three steps, you can do this Not done after one prayer? Just repeat the process...

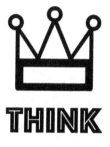

THINK

* Deal with you first. Think the right things about your Father, about faith, and about healing...

* Make sure they think the right things to... affirm and confess to them what you believe. They will "piggy back" on your faith! You set the tone!

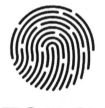

TOUCH

* Touch them. Touch them. And then touch them again.

* As you reach for the oils, explain to them what you are doing, a little about the oils (i.e., Jesus sent the disciples to anoint, James told the early church leaders to do so, etc...), and ask if you may anoint them...

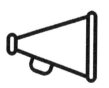

TELL

* Tell them the truth about who they are (removing bad roots and planting good roots).

* Pray- or even command- the sickness to leave.

* Tell them, again, of who pleased the Father is with them and how much they are loved...

* Ask them if they're better- if they're not 100%, pray again... and again!

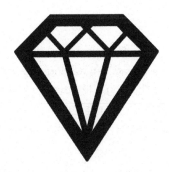

Apply the Steps & Heal

AN ENVIRONMENT OF EASE & EXPECTATION
LEVELS OF ANOINTING
STEP-BY-STEP

☐ What does Paul mean when he preaches that "God is not served by human hands"? How, then, do we "serve" God?

☐ Over the past two years, I've learned firsthand that you can't out-serve or out-minister the physical body you're in. In other words, the "container" you're in must be kept healthy and whole. Face it: no matter how incredible of a destiny you have, you can't experience it if you're sick on the couch. What do you think about this?

APPLY THE STEPS & HEAL

☐ When you were young, you practiced walking... and you fell... a lot! In this chapter we discussed how healing is like this. It's a gift *and* a skill. It's an ability God gives and it's something we can actually get better at doing. In what ways does this are you to actually "try it"? In what ways does this might you nervous?

☐ Review the *Direction-Action-Miracle* concept presented in this chapter. Every time Jesus gave a *direction*, the people who took *action* experienced a *miracle*. For instance, Jesus told the servants at the Wedding at Cana of Galilee to fill the water pots with water (John 2:1f.). They did (*direction-action-miracle*) and He made new wine. He commanded Mary & Martha to roll the stone away from Lazarus' tomb (John 11:1f.). They did (*direction-action-miracle*) and Lazarus came forth! Where else in the Bible do you see this pattern? Now, what *direction* are you receiving? What *action* do you need to take? What *miracle* to you expect to see?

☐ Let's discuss the position you pray from. You are praying *from* the Kingdom and *from* victory- not *from* earth *for* victory. What does it mean that...

- You pray with authority...?

- You pray *from* victory instead of *for* victory...?

- You pray, joining something that is already happening...

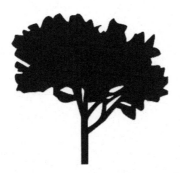

Appendix

Keep Moving!

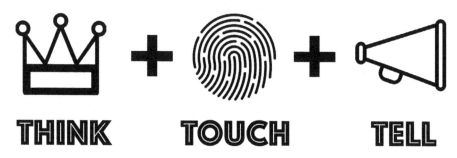

THINK

* Review the Scripture and the 3 habits

TOUCH

* Get the tools you need- the oils, online materials, supplemental resources…

TELL

* Do it. Practice. Get experience… you'll get better & better with time!

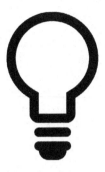

Helpful Resources
TOOLS TO HELP YOU GROW

To learn the theology (think)

The Healing Workshop- the online class- go to www.TheHealingWorkshop.info for more info

The Overflow Podcast- go to Jenkins.tv for episodes

From Slavery to Sonship, Jack Frost (book)

Grace Basics (8-part online video class)- FREE with purchase of the *Think, Touch, Tell* online class- available as a stand alone at www.GraceBasics.info.

The Kingdom 101: Living Under and Open Heaven (Andrew Edwin Jenkins)

Power Healing, John Wimber (book)

To learn the products (touch)

See the free video courses available at www.overflowfaith.com/p/the-healing-sessions.

Healing Oils of the Bible, Dr. David Stewart (book)

Must Haves for Wellness (online video class)- FREE with purchase of the *Think, Touch, Tell* online class

Essential Oil Pocket Reference (Life Science Publishing) (book)

To learn the practice of healing (tell)

"Laying on of hands," document and video- which explores this practice and the doctrine of impartation

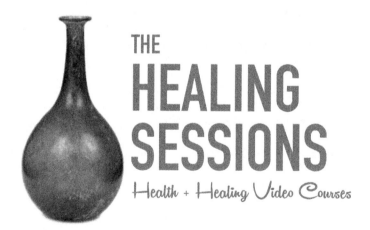

THE
HEALING
SESSIONS
Health + Healing Video Courses

Go to www.overflowfaith.com/p/the-healing-sessions for free, instant access.

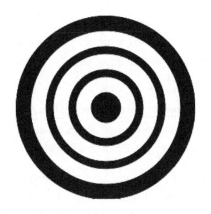

Start Your Own

YOUR HEALING MINISTRY IS AS EASY AS THINK, TOUCH, TELL!

Here's an easy on-ramp to starting your own healing ministry. This may be something you do on your own, something you start as a stand-alone ministry, a small group you lead, a ministry you lead at your church with the blessing of your pastor, or some other way you see fit to do this.

Step 1: Think

First, get the information. That way, you can review the info, you can continue learning, and you can equip yourself to even teach others.

This curriculum is available as an online class, *complete with multiple videos on each of the lessons, as well as the entire eBoo*k. Everything you need to get started is there.

- **Step-by-step training** to get you learn how to lead a team, bless others, have some of the most fun you will ever have, while making an eternal difference that changes people's lives now in a measurable way!

- **Access to the online support groups!** You'll see what others are doing, what they're learning in the process, and learn from people actually involved in helping others (Priceless)

- **FREE** ticket to the next live workshop! ($97 value). You can use the ticket provided to sit in, bringing this book with you, or you can pay a nominal materials fee and receive an additional book at the door.

> FIRST, GET THE INFORMATION. THAT WAY, YOU CAN REVIEW THE INFO, YOU CAN CONTINUE LEARNING, AND YOU CAN EQUIP YOURSELF TO EVEN TEACH OTHERS.

- **FREE** *The Kingdom 101* eBook (600-plus pages where we walk through the theology of grace, as well as the practical application of ministering from grace). This is a must have book that takes many of the concepts presented in this training material even deeper! ($27 value)

- **FREE** document, "Laying on of hands," which explores this practice and the doctrine of impartation with a FREE video teaching on the topic ($97 value)

- **FREE** *Grace Basics* video series. This 8-part teaching series walks you through the foundational beliefs behind Think, Touch, Tell. You'll learn more about who God is, your new nature that is recreated into Christ's image, understand the importance of focusing on the Savior instead of sin, and learn the proper place of the Law and confession in the life of a believer! ($37 value)

- **FREE** *Must Haves for Wellness* video class. This 10-part series will show you two ways to get healing oils and other great wellness products FREE every single month. ($47 value)

You'll also receive a few tools that will help you teach this material to others:

- **BONUS!**- Images of all of the slides we use in the videos and in the live workshops ($87 value)

- **BONUS!**- Downloadable versions of all of our charts, graphs, and hand-outs that you've seen throughout this book (that way you can just press "print" instead of having to find a copy machine!). ($27 value)

Yes- that's over $400 of added bonuses to the material!!!

Be sure to use the coupon code HEALING (in all caps) to get a HUGE SAVINGS on the online version of this class!

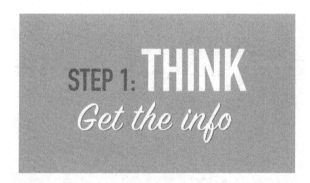

Step 2: Touch

Second, you need to acquire the tools to get started. We suggest you order Young Living's Premium Starter Kit (it's an amazing value- it comes with 11 essential oils, a diffuser, and several other items!). You will eventually want the *Twelve Oils of Ancient Scripture* package, too.

If you're able to acquire these at the same time, do so! If not, order the Premium Starter Kit right away- and set an Essential Rewards order for the *Twelve Oils of*

Ancient Scripture to come to you next month. (Essential Rewards is a non-obligation, non-contract program that gives you discounted shipping and points back which you can use for free products. We don't buy anything unless we do it on this program- we love free stuff!).

> SECOND, YOU NEED TO ACQUIRE THE TOOLS TO GET STARTED.

If you're waiting to get the *Twelve Oils of Ancient Scripture* (you'll want to order the other kit *first*, so that you receive the 24% discount on the Twelve Oils kit!), place it on Essential Rewards now and it will ship in approximately 30 days, giving you time to learn the first set of oils. (By placing the order on Essential Rewards, you earn points towards future *free* products!)

To place your order, consult with the person who gave you this material if they are a business-building distributor with Young Living Essential Oils. You will need their coupon code to receive the wholesale discount!

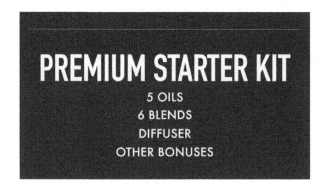

PREMIUM STARTER KIT
5 OILS
6 BLENDS
DIFFUSER
OTHER BONUSES

If they are not a distributor OR if you found this info on your own, ***please go to YoungLiving.com, click "Become a Member," and use the Enroller / Sponsor ID 1481259 (Overflow, LLC). That will place you on our team!***

By the way, email us a copy of your receipt to AJ@overflow.org and I'll send you a link for FREE ACCESS to an online version of the class recorded just for team members like you.

STEP 2: TOUCH
Get the tools

Step 3: Tell

Third, you must communicate the information and begin touching others with healing. There are a few ways you can do this.

- **You can lead a workshop.**

    - You'll need a book for each participant, which you can order on our website. We suggest you order them a few weeks in advance, to insure they arrive on time.

> THIRD, YOU MUST COMMUNICATE THE INFORMATION AND BEGIN TOUCHING OTHERS WITH HEALING.

    - You'll find the slides in the online version of the class.

    - Not ready to teach it yourself? Grab the videos online and "press play" for your group!

    - If a 3-hour or 4-hour workshop seems a bit daunting, consider spreading the information over the course of a few weeks. Teach one topic a week.

- **You can schedule an event.** To schedule a healing workshop, call 205-291-1391. Or email AJ@overflow.org.

Whatever you decide, *your time is now!* Jesus empowered you to do this!

STEP 3: **TELL**
Do it!

Answer Key

GET THE ANSWERS HERE

1. Intro

A. Heaven

1. Heaven coming down

2. tree of life

3. Kingdom, don't, old identity

B. Healing, wholeness, Healing, wholeness, Health, wellness

1. food, more

2. healing, wholeness

C. simple strategy

1. think, touch, tell

2. important

3. specific actions, wholeness, healing

2. Habit 1 = Think

A. who God is

1. the Father

2. plainly, means

3. big leap

4. radical difference

B. faith

1. work, claim, healing

2. formula, box, fit

C. healing

1. foundational concepts

2. three, healing, two

3. *iaomai*

4. *therapeuo*, natural means

5. both, Jesus'

6. healing

7. two kinds

8. choose life, live well

9. *sozo*, total healing

10. scope, depth, today

11. forgiveness, restoration, reconciliation

12. forgiveness of sins
13. practical application

3. Habit 2 = Touch
A. Essential oils
1. power to heal
2. healing properties
3. essential oils, relevant
4. essential oils, ministry
5. lot, several important
6. healing power
B. explained
1. other oils
2. aromatic, volatile, life source, essence
3. grades, qualities
4. Quality, Biblical anointing
5. How, why
6. touching, breathing, swallowing
7. throughout, Bible
C. higher, faster
1. frequency, frequency, electrical energy
2. frequency, health, alive
3. modern medicine
4. above the line

4. The Oils
A. need
1. your body
2. see
B. Premium Starter Kit
1. Premium Starter Kit
2. starter kit
C. twelve, Scripture
1. entire person
2. reflexology, thought
3. basics, oils, Bible

5. Habit 3 = Tell
A. body, soul, spirit
1. spirit, body, deepest, inside out

2. spirit, body

B. presence, power

1. different

2. nickels, noses, seats, money, give

3. Christ's

4. you, everything

C. right

1. frequency, higher

2. healing, everything

3. salvation, *sozo*, Savior

4. Father, bless

5. bad fruit, healthy root

6. Next Steps

A. you

1. to you, through you

2. underlying beliefs

3. health, *therapeuo*

4. through people

B. Review, learned

C. tools, successful

7. Step-by-Step Ministry Model

A. beliefs, behaviors

1. to you, through you

2. skill, confidence, do it

B. anointing, heal

1. better

2. healed, healing

C. healing, wholeness

1. stand

2. barriers

3. carry, barrier

4. build your case, supports your request

5. call it, claim it, command it

6. action

7. present, stand in

8. *therapeuo*, now

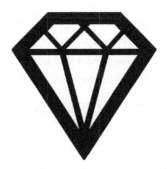

Bio
WHO WE ARE

I'm a thinker, a writer, a teacher... a guy who's led in churches and nonprofits, a guy who's preached and taught and done a bunch of other stuff, too. I've been overwhelmed by my Father's grace.

We've been married seventeen years and have nine kids. The two most common questions we get are:

- "Are they all yours?" (meaning, ours together- or were some hers and some mine and then we got married. Answer: They are all "ours together"- Seven biological and two are adopted from Uganda. *And,*

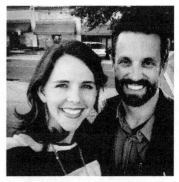

With Cristy at one of our favorite restaurants- on the weekly date night!

- "Have you figured out what causes it?" (or, some version of that, i.e., Do you have a TV?, etc.). Answer: What do you think? Do you think we've figured it out?

BIO

The kids are incredible. They pray, they serve, they love doing ministry. And, of course (since they're kids), they love swashbuckling, too. FYI, they always get a prize when they're in public and someone remarks about how well behaved they are, so throw them a bone next time you see them. They'll never forget you. I promise.

Our kids' ages range from 17 down to 4. Besides these, another precious one is in heaven.

They're quite diverse:

- A budding author who likes to sing and and create her own books and films!

- A tender young lady who is nurturing, kind and an amazing gymnast + volleyball player + anything else she decides to do (she brought home some hardware from her first meet!). She's also known as our faith healer (no kidding).

- A young boy who loves to preach, has mastered Legos, and shoots his own videos in his spare time.

- Another young boy who is tender and compassionate- and will drop whatever he's doing to help you.

- A young boy who is genuine, smiles constantly and loves people- and people love him. "I'm the fun one," he muses.

- Another boy who is larger than life and can out-dance anyone. Period.

- The Sweet (self-explanatory, especially after you meet him and listen to his buttery voice).

- The youngest girl, we affectionately call "Mini"- not to be confused with her determination and perseverance, though. *And,*

- *Turbo*- no explanation needed.

Yep, that's 6 boys and 3 girls!

BIO

Most of what we do, we do together. You'll see us (together) doing various service projects around our city, riding bikes at the park, hiking at Ruffner Mountain, staying up 'til midnight for a "movie night" (the kids' favorite- the way they count in all birthdays, holidays, and anything else you can think of), or going on some other adventure.

So, that's my highlight reel. Thanks for your interest in the book. If you have questions, comments, or just want to connect, you can find me online at www.WeOverflow.com, or via email: AndrewEJenkins@mac.com. And, yes, I'm on Facebook and Twitter and everything else!

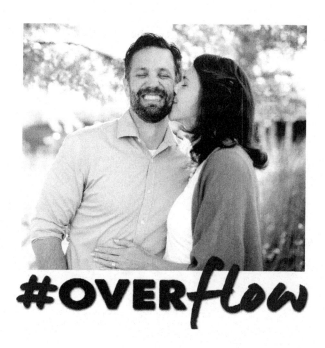

If Jesus healed everyone

and if He said we would do greater things than He did

WHY ISN'T EVERYONE HEALED TODAY?

If you...

- Believe healing power is available today and feel like God has tapped you to share His abundance & provision with others...

- Want a step-by-step process that's backed by the Bible, history, and science...

- Would love to give yourself and the people you love options when the miracles seem just out of reach...

- Think experiencing the Father's heart would be fun and invigorating...

Then this book is just for you!

34483515R00146

Made in the USA
Middletown, DE
27 January 2019